Solving America's Healthcare Crisis

**powerful information that will
change your life;
join the revolution that is reforming
America's healthcare system!**

by Pamela A. Popper, Ph.D., N.D.

This book has been written and published strictly for informational purposes only and in no way should it be used as a substitute for recommendations from your own health care practitioner. All of the facts in this book came from medical files, clinical journals, scientific publications, personal interviews, published trade books, magazine articles and the personal practice experiences of the authorities quoted or the sources cited. You should not consider the educational material herein to be the practice of medicine or to replace consultation with a physician or other practitioner. The author and publisher of this information are providing you with this information in order that you can have knowledge. You can choose, at your own risk, to act on that knowledge.

Published by:
PB Industries, Inc.
510 East Wilson Bridge Road Suite G
Worthington,Ohio 43085
614 841-7700
614 841-7703 fax
800 761-8210 US only

Health care professionals like dietitians and doctors are licensed by the states in which they live and practice. Professional associations like the American Medical Association and the American Dietetic Association have helped to pass laws in many states that prevent other competing groups from practicing. Not only is the information most consumers are getting about diet, health, and medical care inaccurate, but careful control of which types of people are permitted to discuss these topics is maintained by a relatively small group of individuals who are financially supported by food and drug companies and have an interest in maintaining the status quo.

All of this adds up to a terribly misinformed public that gets sicker instead of better and spends an ever-increasing amount of money while doing so.

When the health insurance reform bill passed in 2010, many people thought that this was a step in the right direction in improving America's health. I disagree; the law is entirely about who is going to pay for more people to have access to our existing health care system. There are no meaningful provisions for examining the type of health care that Americans are receiving and eliminating those tests and treatments that are not effective. Paying for health care that does not work for millions more people will not solve our health care problem; it will make it worse.

In spite of this, I am optimistic. Things have slowly started to improve, and the reason I have written this book is to accelerate the pace of change. We are about to experience a revolution in health care in America, and this book is designed to help you to learn the truth about diet, health, and medical care so that you can become an active participant in this revolution.

A growing number of doctors are teaching their patients to change their health status through the use of a very specific diet. These doctors are producing results that are nothing short of spectacular. Not only are the results better (disease progression is being stopped and in many cases, diseases are being reversed), but these results are being achieved for a fraction of the cost of drugs and surgery. In this book, you'll read about the scientific research showing that this diet is effective for preventing, stopping the progression of, and reversing many common degenerative diseases. You'll also read about how ineffective traditional medical care, which includes annual exams, diagnostic testing to detect disease in its earliest stages, and most drugs and procedures, really is.

If you're like me, this information is likely to make you angry. You'll be angry that you've been lied to about diet and health. You might be angry about some of the tests, drugs, and procedures to which you or members of your family or your friends have been subjected. You may be angry because the solution to so many of our health care issues has been known for so long and yet is still not generally known. You may even be angry because family members or friends have died who might still be with you if they had access to this information. The key to changing the system is for you to channel that anger into doing something productive.

The first step is to use the information in this book to help you and your family to achieve optimal health. Once you have done so, you can then become a center of influence for your friends and community. You can join us in teaching these concepts to others. You can help up to work on improving school food and children's health. You can join a growing number of people who collectively can overwhelm our existing political system by voting for state and federal officials who will support the dissemination of truthful information, promote meaningful regulation, and the rights of Americans to choose their health care providers and methods of care.

You can also join us in using our collective purchasing power to reward people, companies, organizations, and institutions that support health-promoting foods and medical care, and to starve out those that don't. Using the power of our checkbooks, we can refuse to purchase products from manufacturers of unhealthy foods and factory farms, we can withdraw our support of non-profit organizations that promote ineffective diagnostic tests and treatments, and stop seeing health care practitioners who do not make people well.

Entire governments have been toppled by relatively small groups of people who share a common vision; a strong conviction; and the willingness to fight for the right ideas. I am confident that our current health care system is going to be overthrown in a similar manner. It's time to join this movement and help to accelerate the momentum. Together we can and will change the system and create a healthier America.

Introduction

I did not start my adult life as a health care professional; I did not even consider it as a potential occupation as a young person. In fact, I was one of those people who didn't know what I wanted to be when I grew up. I envied my friends who had decided in high school to be teachers, doctors and lawyers, and hoped that by the time I graduated from high school I would feel inspired to do something. I wasn't.

So I wandered from thing to thing, dabbling in this and that. I spent almost a year in college as a theater major, then changed to piano performance. After two years, I decided I didn't want to play the piano or teach, so I dropped out of school and started a career in sales. I started a business that came to an unfortunate end in 1988, and returned to sales and sales training.

I was good at some of the things I did, but my heart really wasn't in any of them. They were a means to an end, which was to make money and take care of my family.

My only interest in nutrition was in doing whatever it took to stay thin. I took dance lessons as a kid, danced with a local company, and actually owned a dance studio while I was in high school. Dancers were thin, and so thin was what I wanted to be. I learned that the best way to accomplish this goal was to not eat and to smoke cigarettes.

I have never applied moderation to anything I've done. I'm either immersed in something completely or not interested at all, a personality trait which I applied to smoking – I smoked four packs of cigarettes a day. My eating habits were just as abominable. I lived on cookies and coffee; sometimes as much as three pots of coffee per day. I remember being described as "energetic;" I now know I spent a couple of decades just buzzed on caffeine and sugar.

I stopped dancing after high school, and I became completely sedentary. I would place my garbage cans on the hood of my car and drive them to the street; this was one way of many ways I devised in order to avoid physical activity. Once in a while inspiration would hit me and I would join a gym – it seemed like

11

the fashionable thing to do - but I never stuck with an exercise routine for very long. I was busy working and doing other things.

The bottom line is that I was the last person in the world who might be expected to develop a career, and a personal life, that revolved around teaching other people how to eat and exercise.

In 1993, I accidentally happened upon some articles about nutrition and health that indicated that diet might have a profound influence on health. I was curious. I didn't have health problems (that I knew of), but I knew my diet was terrible. I was tired all the time and seemed to be looking older by the day.

An acquaintance recommended that I read a book written by John McDougall, a doctor in California who had been reversing degenerative conditions like heart disease and diabetes with a plant-based diet for 25 years. I couldn't put the book down and stayed up all night reading it. I was astounded at the power of a plant-based diet and equally astounded that I had heard nothing about this before.

Excited at this new discovery, I read other books by Dr. McDougall and then saw the movie *Diet for a New America* produced by John Robbins, which discussed the effects of the traditional Western diet on health and the environment. This was my first exposure to Dr. T. Colin Campbell; the film included an interview with him about The China Project. Subsequently, I also found out about the work of Dr. Neal Barnard, Dr. Caldwell Esselstyn, and others who I talk about and refer to in this book. I continued to be amazed at what I was learning about the diet/health connection.

By this time, I was inspired, excited and I had finally (at the age of 38) figured out what I wanted to be when I grew up! Nutrition was my passion; I wanted to think about it, read about it, and tell everyone else about it 24 hours a day. While I was conducting my informal research, I adopted a plant-based diet (I ate fish a couple of times per month for a few years and then eventually stopped). My physical appearance changed rapidly – I lost weight and body fat, my skin looked great and my energy levels improved significantly. I was learning from personal experience that there really was something powerful about plant-based nutrition.

I knew that in order to be taken seriously, I needed to pursue education in the nutrition field, and became very disappointed when I started looking into my options. Our local university offered a nutrition degree that led to becoming a registered dietitian. But the coursework included a lot of food service curriculum, and an internship for 900 hours that was almost certain to involve institutional food cookery. I looked into alternatives, which were marginally better. These programs, many of which were offered through distance learning, offered more science, but emphasized the use of supplements, bio-individuality, and other concepts I had already learned were incorrect. The most disappointing thing of all for me was that none of the nutrition programs I investigated really taught diet as a preventive or healing tool; none of them focused on the work of professionals like Dr. John McDougall and Dr. T. Colin Campbell.

I chose the best of the less-than-optimal options for me and made up my mind to do whatever it took to get through school, even though I disagreed with the underlying philosophy of most of what I was being taught. I encountered a similar set of choices later when I chose to become a naturopath. I did not want to be a traditional doctor, dispensing drugs and performing surgery (options that mitigate symptoms but do not address the underlying cause of disease). Training for naturopaths does emphasize diet and lifestyle, but focuses on the use of dietary supplements, herbs, and other more "natural" treatments to mitigate symptoms. These treatments are less toxic, but still do not address the underlying cause of disease. Naturopathy was closer to my anticipated scope of practice, so I pursued that degree, but again, it was not a great choice, just the better of the not so great options.

My evaluation of educational opportunities helped me to understand that health care professionals are really victims of their training. Most people enter the healing arts because they want to help people. They invest years of their lives in training, which is quite expensive in most cases. It is not their fault that medical and health care education doesn't stress the importance of diet and its use as an intervention tool. I am lucky that I learned about the efficacy of a plant-based diet from the right practitioners *before* my journey into health care began, or my career path would have definitely been quite different.

When I started my education, I didn't have a business plan in mind. I just wanted to learn about nutrition and health. The Wellness Forum started quite accidentally. My friends and acquaintances were curious about what I was learning and were constantly asking questions. I was, frankly, surprised at the level of interest. I organized a small class in my home in September 1996, to share what I knew about nutrition. Twelve people attended. There were no curriculum books (this was really informal), but they liked it - and asked if we could meet again the following week. They brought friends and pretty soon my house was a very busy place. Within a short time, both my neighbors and my family were ready for me to teach somewhere else, so I rented a small office close to my house and started holding classes regularly. In the beginning, I didn't even charge people, and hoped that when I started charging the people would continue to attend (they did!). And so, The Wellness Forum was launched.

Over a period of time, I became amazed at the results people were achieving as they ate less animal food and more plant food. They lost weight easily. Their skin cleared up. Aches and pains started to go away. We were really not promising people outcomes in those days, but our students came to classes anxious to share their stories. I became more and more excited, and the more I learned, the more convinced I became that this message needed to be delivered to everyone.

I had no plan for employing other people, but excited people who experienced health improvement and weight loss wanted to help. Locally, some members asked if they could teach classes. By this time, we had an informal curriculum that others could follow, so I began to let others teach. A good friend, Dr. Jane Powley, agreed to open the first remote location in Wilmington Delaware, and shortly after, another good friend, Sue Scharf, opened a location in Grand Rapids, Michigan. Other healthy graduates came forward and became the first employees of The Wellness Forum. One successful program graduate, Gary Morse, started working a few hours per week and now runs our entire operation as general manager. I cannot emphasize how important these people became to our growing success story; I could never have done this by myself.

I think what attracted these great people to The Wellness Forum and what kept them engaged, even through the early days of chaos, was the feeling that we had stumbled upon something great; that we were making positive change. Everyone longs to be part of a great cause, and I think The Wellness Forum has always been more of a cause than a business. In fact, in the early days during one of our informal meetings in my family room, we were talking about our goals for the future and actually committed to paper the goal to "change health care in America." I don't think any of us knew what that really would entail, but those commitments definitely inspired us to work hard!

What continues to fuel our enthusiasm and the company's growth is the results we see every day. People who have suffered from gastrointestinal disorders for years are able to stop taking their drugs and no longer spend six to eight weeks per year in the hospital. People with high cholesterol and cardiovascular disease are able to discontinue medications and avoid surgery. People with type 2 diabetes get rid of it. The thing that amazes me is that I am just as excited about every success story today as I was years ago when this all started!

By far, however, the most rewarding stories come from women who have suffered from infertility or have had several miscarriages and desperately want to have children. Although it makes sense that nutrition and health status would affect the ability to conceive and carry a child to term, it never occurred to me that our plant-based diet could be the key to helping these women. And there are just so many. About one third of American couples are dealing with infertility today, and many of them are mortgaging their houses and cashing in their retirement funds to pay for expensive fertility treatments.

In the early days, we had reports from women who became pregnant after changing their diets, and eventually we determined that this was a fairly predictable result when women adopted a plant-based diet. To date, we have helped over 100 women to have babies who were told that they most likely would not. These include women who have undergone treatment for cancer that resulted in early menopause, women who had four or more miscarriages, women who had stopped ovulating years before they became Wellness Forum members, and other amazing stories.

We call these babies "Wellness Forum babies" and we are as excited (well almost as excited) as their families are when they are born! I cry every time someone sends me a picture, and it motivates me to do even more to spread the world about this diet.

During the last 18 years, my weight, appearance and health status have improved – some people say I look younger now than I did 18 years ago. One person even asked if I had a face lift (I have not). I love being healthy and looking and feeling great, but another important transformation for me was my in my professional life. Sixteen years ago, I worked because I had to and I did well because it was expected of me. I had learned to "bloom where I was planted" and make the most of the things I did for a living, so I tried to enjoy them as much as possible. I've generally been a happy person, even when life was not entirely going my way.

Today, however, things have changed. I LOVE what I do. I cannot imagine a life without The Wellness Forum or one that does not involve the work that we do, helping people change their lives through plant-based nutrition. People accuse me of being a workaholic, but I remind them of the Will Rogers quote, "The finest day in a man's life is when he falls in love with his work, because then he never has to go to work again." This is not a job; it's my passion and what makes me want to get up in the morning. If there were more hours in the day, I would spend them on this! One great thing about practicing dietary excellence and optimal habits is that I can look forward to helping people to regain and maintain their health for decades more! I don't want to retire; I feel like I am just getting started.

Our efforts to educate the public about plant-based nutrition are gaining momentum, and one of the reasons is that those of us who are doing this type of work have connected with one another and are working together. I feel incredibly honored to be a part of this group.

As I mentioned earlier, I read books and articles written by plant-based health care gurus like John McDougall, Neal Barnard, Caldwell Esselstyn and Colin Campbell. I used to dream about meeting these people someday, and it is an unbelievable privilege to now be working with them side by side. I wake up every day grateful that this is not a dream; that it really is my real life. And I have more determination than ever to get this message out to the masses.

The State of American Health

The most important part of this mission statement is "empower individuals to take control of their health." The first step in learning how to achieve optimum health is learning that it is not your insurance company's responsibility to keep you healthy; it is also not the federal government's job, or even your doctor's job to keep you healthy – it is yours! I certainly don't want to imply that these institutions or individuals do not care about you at all. But the bottom line is that you have the biggest vested interest in what happens to you from a health perspective, so you have to be in charge.

My friend Dr. Isadore Rosenfeld, a doctor who believes in patients making informed choices, has often said "An educated patient gets the best medical care." While I agree with this, I take it a step further – "An educated patient requires *less* medical care." And that should be your goal – do your best to reduce your need for medical services. Stay out of the doctor's office and hospital if at all possible by taking care of yourself.

It is important to clarify an important point. I am not suggesting that all drug treatments and Western approaches to dealing with illness should be avoided. In fact, there are some aspects of our medical system that are the best on the planet. Our diagnostic capability, for example, is awesome, and Western medicine is the best at emergency intervention and trauma.

But Western medicine has been miserably ineffective in preventing, stopping the progression of, and reversing degenerative disease. The first method of treatment is usually drugs, which suppress symptoms rather than addressing the underlying problem. Drugs and surgery should be "last resorts"

19

to be used when less toxic and invasive treatments such as nutrition, exercise, and lifestyle choices have been exhausted.

It is time for our medical system to approach health differently. Financially we can't afford not to. Our health care system is a major factor in America's growing financial crisis. Our health care budget has ballooned to over $2.2 trillion dollars.[1] We are spending $174 billion annually on diabetes,[2] $475 billion on heart disease and stroke,[3] $174 billion on complications from obesity,[4] and $228.1 billion on cancer.[5] The good news is that 85% of these costs are for chronic, degenerative conditions, most of which are preventable, and many of which are reversible by changing our diet and lifestyle habits.

Even more important than the financial pressures we are enduring as a result of all of this illness is the decreased quality of life experienced by many adults. Today, 23.6 million Americans have diabetes,[6] there are 57 million pre-diabetics[7] who will most certainly become diabetic if they do not change their ways; 80 million Americans have at least one marker for coronary artery disease;[8] and every day 1500 Americans die from cancer.[9]

The most frightening health statistic is that the average age at which people are developing these problems continues to go down. Our children are now developing diseases formerly associated with older adults. In 2008, the American Academy of Pediatrics recommended that children with a family history of heart disease be tested for cholesterol before the age of ten. The AAP also recommended that children with high cholesterol be given statin medications.[10] So many children are being diagnosed with type 2 diabetes that we no longer refer to it as "adult onset type 2 diabetes," and instead just call it "type 2 diabetes."

The ramifications of people developing more serious illnesses at an earlier age are huge. The expense of administering traditional health care, meaning drugs and surgeries, for the greater part of a lifetime for millions of Americans, is beyond our financial capability. But the quality of life issues are even more serious. Life is not easy while taking drugs with sometimes very serious

Nutritional Confusion

Nutritionally confused? You're not alone. A great debate takes place daily among medical professionals about the best diet for humans. Many of these professionals are doctors and others with impressive credentials; yet they dispense information in direct contradiction with one another. It is very hard for the average consumer to sort out.

What accounts for so many supposedly qualified people offering such diverse advice? Interest in diet and health has never been greater in the U.S. than it is today. There are millions of dollars to be made by writing a book about diet that is different, works faster, has a unique angle, or offers the key to health, weight loss, or anti-aging. Thus we see books about how to eat like a hunter/gatherer (even though none of us are hunter/gatherers!); how to eat based on your blood type, your body type or your metabolic type; how to lose weight without changing your diet at all; and how to reverse aging with special supplements. It is almost certain that some books become popular essentially because they give people permission to eat lobster in butter sauce, cheese, meat, and fat, which appeals to more people than advice to eat more fruit and vegetables.

Many of today's popular programs and books are not based on research and science, but rather stories. The authors tell *stories* of people who have thrived by following their advice, but they often do not present or cite research to back their claims. Stories are interesting, and there are some stories to illustrate points in this book, but they should never be relied on exclusively when making important decisions about diet and health. For example, people often tell stories about a relative who ate bacon, eggs and cheese three times a day, lived to be 95 years old, and died in his sleep. The story may be true, but scientific studies show that this is not a likely outcome for most people consuming a similar diet.

Another limitation of many popular books and programs is that they promise short-term results without considering long-term ramifications for health. These programs become popular because they "work." This is especially true with weight-loss programs, and high-protein diets are a good example. These diets *do* work, but they are health-destroying in the long term. If the criteria for evaluating a weight loss program are only that "it works," there are many things that work. One is cocaine addiction; in fact, most cocaine addicts are quite skinny! Another is chemotherapy; patients nauseous from treatments often don't feel like eating and they lose weight. But no one in their right mind would suggest that people start using cocaine or undergoing chemotherapy in order to lose weight because we all know that in the long run these are not health-promoting programs.

It is important to consider not only short-term results, but long-term health consequences when evaluating diet, weight loss, and health improvement strategies. The research relied upon to make the recommendations in this book are based on long-term observations of the effects of varying diets on health. For example, Dr. Caldwell Esselstyn at The Cleveland Clinic placed his cardiovascular patients on a diet to reverse their disease and followed his original patient group for 12 years. Dr. Roy Swank followed his original group of multiple sclerosis patients for 34 years. This is a very important distinction.

But an even bigger issue affecting the advice being given to Americans daily is the way in which nutrition policies and dietary guidelines are developed by the U.S. government, and how those policies are then used by government agencies, national health organizations, and health care professionals to deliver recommendations to Americans about how to eat.

The USDA and Dietary Recommendations

President Abraham Lincoln signed legislation passed by Congress that called for the formation of The United States Department of Agriculture (USDA) in 1862. The USDA was chartered as an advocacy organization for farmers, and even today the agency's written information focuses on its relationship to agriculture.[13] In fact, the USDA's mandate originally was to "Test by experiment the use of agricultural implements and the value of seeds, soils, manures and animals; undertake the chemical investigation of soils, grains, fruits, vegetables and manures, publishing the results."[14] Since agriculture is a vital part of our economy and important for our very survival, having a government agency dedicated to helping farmers is probably a good idea.

But the problem is that the USDA is also charged with developing nutritional guidelines for Americans. These recommendations are not only communicated directly to the American public, but are also used as a basis for labeling processed and packaged foods; for the development of parameters for school lunches; for determining which foods will be made available under the WIC (Women, Infants and Children) program; as a basis for training many nutrition professionals, and for the design of curricula used to teach children about nutrition in public school classrooms.

This presents an institutional conflict of interest for the USDA. How can a federal agency charged with helping farmers also be charged with developing nutritional recommendations for Americans? How can this organization ever tell people to reduce the consumption of or eliminate a food produced profitably by the very farmers it is supposed to help? In my opinion, assistance for farmers and the development of nutritional recommendations for Americans should be administered by two separate agencies.

Inaccurate USDA Guidelines

The first USDA dietary recommendations were developed by Wilbur Atwater, an agricultural chemist, in 1894.[15]   Vitamins and minerals had not yet been discovered, so Atwater's recommendations focused on making sure people consumed enough calories daily, with an emphasis on eating more protein, beans and vegetables, and less fat, sugar and starchy foods. These weren't the worst recommendations issued by the USDA, but they did over-emphasize the importance of protein, while limiting certain plant foods like rice and potatoes, the foundation of the diets of some of the healthiest people on the planet. Atwater had conducted no research on the relationship of varying diets and health; he had merely observed the eating habits of various groups of people in the U.S. in developing his recommendations.

The first official USDA Food Guide, *How to Select Foods,* was

27

published in 1916.[16] Written by Caroline Hunt, a nutritionist for the USDA and the first professor of Home Economics at the University of Wisconsin, this was the first time guidelines were based on food groups, a format that is still used by the agency today. The five food groups recommended by Hunt were:
1. Milk and meat
2. Cereals
3. Vegetables and fruit
4. Fats and fatty foods
5. Sugars and sugary foods

In the early 1940's, the National Academy of Sciences formed the Food and Nutrition Board, which established the Recommended Daily Allowances for calories and for eight nutrients. The USDA was then charged with developing dietary recommendations that met the standards established by the Food and Nutrition Board.

In 1946, the first recommendations issued based on these new guidelines, the National Nutrition Guide,[17] were published. The number of food groups was expanded from five to seven:
1. Milk and milk products
2. Meat, poultry, fish, eggs, beans, peas, and nuts
3. Bread, flour and cereals
4. Leafy green and yellow vegetables
5. Potatoes and sweet potatoes
6. Citrus, tomato, cabbage, and salad greens
7. Butter and fortified margarine

In 1956 the number of food groups was condensed to four;[18] milk, meat, fruits and vegetables, and grain products. For the first time, serving sizes were included. Over the years, more food groups were added, and eventually the now-familiar food pyramid was adopted. This design included 6 food groups, and the number of daily recommended servings of each:

Breads, cereals, rice and pasta
Vegetable group
Fruit group
Milk, yogurt and cheese
Meat, poultry, fish, eggs, dry beans and nuts
Fats, oils and sweets

Today, the USDA, in conjunction with the Department of Health and Human Services, issues a new set of dietary guidelines based on recommendations from a Federal Dietary Guidelines Advisory Committee, which is convened every five years. This committee is supposed to be comprised of experts appointed by government officials, but often these experts have financial ties to agricultural organizations and food manufacturers. In 1999, the Physicians Committee for Responsible Medicine in Washington, D.C. obtained information from the USDA showing that six out of the eleven members of the committee revising the guidelines at that time had financial ties to the meat, dairy and egg industries.[19]

Agricultural groups and food producers understand clearly that national food policies affect their sales. They aggressively and successfully influence the development of dietary guidelines by presenting promotional information about their products at advisory committee meetings. They also lobby Congress to prevent the dispensing of nutritional advice that might suggest that Americans eat less of the products they produce. Many of these groups, particularly those that represent the interests of beef and dairy producers, are extremely well-funded.[20] Thus Americans continue to get nutrition information based on the influence of lobbying groups, not scientific research on diet and health.

The USDA Promotes an Animal Foods-Based Diet

The USDA uses many methods to promote agricultural products to Americans. One important and very well-funded strategy is the "checkoff" program.

The USDA requires dairy producers to contribute 15 cents for every 100 pounds of milk they sell to the dairy checkoff program. In 2005, this program generated $160 million, which was spent on "public education" and marketing. These funds pay for campaigns like the ads featuring celebrities with milk mustaches.

Since the national dairy checkoff program began in 1983, consumption of total milk (the amount of milk that goes into all dairy products)[21] has increased from 522 pounds a year to currently more than 605 pounds a year.

By 2007, the dairy checkoff program had reached $175.2 million for advertising and promotion. Here are a few examples of how this money was invested:[22]

- $26.7 million - Retail – promotion through retailers and branded manufacturers
- $31.6 million - School Marketing – "increases fluid milk and dairy consumption and promotes dairy as part of a healthy lifestyle at our nation's schools"
- $4.0 million – Dairy Ingredient Manufacturing – "works closely with food and beverage manufacturers to increase the use of dairy ingredients"
- $2.0 million - Butter Promotions – "helps promote the use of butter on a national level"
- $14.0 million – Nutrition Affairs – "communicates dairy's role as part of a healthy diet and government recommendations to consume three servings of low- or non-fat dairy products each day"
- $15.5 million – Product and Nutrition Innovation – "conducts research to identify new uses for dairy products that meet consumers' needs, provides assistance in new product development and conducts nutrition research to help advance dairy's role as a key part of a healthy diet"

The USDA even issues reports to Congress about its dairy-promoting activities. The mission of the National Dairy Promotion and Research Board is "to coordinate a promotion and research program that expands domestic and foreign markets for fluid milk, and dairy products produced in the United States."

In 2003, The USDA Report to Congress on Dairy Promotion Programs included information about how the government assisted fast food restaurants like Wendy's and Pizza Hut in increasing cheese consumption by adding it to menu items. Taco Bell introduced a Steak Quesadilla that used eight times more cheese than other items on its menu. Pizza Hut made 2002 the "Summer of Cheese." A 12-week promotion resulted in the sale of 102 million additional pounds of cheese during that summer alone. Wendy's introduced the Cheddar Lovers' Bacon Cheeseburger, and during one four-week period, sold sandwiches that collectively contained 1.5 million additional pounds of cheese.[23] It is ironic that this increased consumption of all of this cheese, filled with saturated fat, was encouraged by a government agency that is supposed to be providing the public with dietary information designed to improve and maintain health.

The dairy industry is not the only food group helped by a checkoff program – the beef and pork industries have checkoff programs too. Unfortunately, there are no big-budget promotional programs for vegetables, fruit, potatoes, or legumes.

Recommendations from
Nutrition Professionals

The USDA is only part of the problem, however. The dietary recommendations issued by the USDA are then used by nutrition professionals, including many dietitians. The American Dietetic Association (ADA) is a national organization that is basically a trade group for dietitians. The organization markets itself and its members as the best resource for Americans to obtain nutrition advice. Dietitians and their national organization should provide the very best science-based recommendations to Americans about diet in order to help people to prevent, stop the progression of, or reverse degenerative disease. There are, indeed, some very good practicing dietitians today, so my statements should not be considered an indictment of all dietitians. But the ADA has financial conflicts of interest that affect its stance on many issues, since it derives a significant portion of its revenue from manufacturing companies and agricultural organizations.

According to its 2008 annual report,[24] the ADA took in $1,888,275 in sponsorship money, $4,126,654 for programs and meetings, and $123,000 in advertising revenue during the previous fiscal year. Coca-Cola, the National Dairy Council and Pepsi-Co are listed as "Partners;" General Mills, Kellogg and Mars, Inc. are listed as "Premier Sponsors;" and "Event Sponsors" include the American Beverage Association and Post Cereals. In return for this support, the organization promotes products grown or made by its contributors.

At varying times during the last several years, I have visited the ADA's website to view "position papers" on various topics. These papers are sponsored by advertisers and have included statements advising people that ice cream is a good source of calcium, and that chewing gum can re-enamelize the teeth. The organization continues to insist that all foods can be included in a healthy diet, and that there are no good or bad foods. This advice pleases sponsors and motivates them to write checks, but contributes to the declining health of Americans, many of whom love to hear that ice cream builds healthy bones

Questionable Advice from "Disease" Groups

National disease groups have similar financial conflicts of interest. For many months the "Health Tip of the Day" on the American Diabetes Association's website was sponsored by Eskimo Pie. This cannot be because anyone actually believes that Eskimo Pies are healthy for diabetics.

The American Heart Association is heavily funded by drug companies and food manufacturers. Its 2009 Annual Report[25] listed Astra Zeneca, Novartis, Merck, Pfizer, Con Agra Foods, and Proctor and Gamble as having made cumulative contributions of over $1,000,000 each. The AHA also operates a certification program which endorses foods with a "heart check mark." The program is paid for by food companies, who are charged on a sliding scale based on the number of products submitted for certification. In February 2010 the "approved" products list included Kansas City Seasoned Beef Steak and Butterball Original Deep-Fried Honey Turkey Roast.[26] The average person with no formal nutrition education most likely knows that these are not heart-healthy foods.

At the same time, on January 4 2010, the AHA's website[27] featured no information about Dr. Caldwell Esselstyn and his dietary program, which has been proven to stop the progression of and even reverse cardiovascular disease, even in patients who were told that they were terminally ill by their expert cardiologists.

It is true that national health organizations are staffed with many well-meaning individuals who want to help sick people. But it is almost impossible to do so while significant portions of revenues are derived from drug and food manufacturers.

The Bottom Line

It is unfortunate, but Americans cannot trust the government, national health organizations, and most health and nutrition professionals to provide reliable and science-based dietary recommendations. It is therefore important to seek information from sources that are not compromised by financial conflicts of interest.

I am very proud of the fact that The Wellness Forum does not take money from food manufacturers, agricultural organizations, lobbyists, or other groups, and therefore can provide objective information about nutrition and healthcare. It's an important reason why I can write a book like this that criticizes so many organizations, companies, health care methods, and practitioners. I don't work for those people or institutions – I work for you and other consumers who want to know the truth about these issues.

The Wellness Forum's

Eating Plan
for
Optimum Health

Humans were designed to eat a whole-foods, plant-based diet, with animal foods, if they are consumed, eaten in tiny quantities as a condiment. We refer to this diet as a program of *dietary excellence.*

The Wellness Forum has developed its own Food Guide Pyramid to reflect the eating habits of the some of the healthiest populations on the planet, and the research of doctors who have carefully documented health improvement using dietary intervention. This pyramid features an eating plan including whole grains, potatoes, legumes, steamed and raw vegetables, and fruit. Nuts and seeds and other high-fat plant foods are condiments; oils and dairy are eliminated; and animal foods are optional.

Consuming ample amounts of foods like rice, beans and potatoes is important because these foods are *filling.* The hunger signal is very powerful - it has kept humans alive for a very long time - and it is only satisfied when the stomach is filled.

Satiety, or a sense of fullness, relies on stretch receptors that send a message to the brain that the stomach is full from enough volume of food; and nutrient receptors that tell the brain that the nutrient density of the food is sufficient. High-fiber foods fill the stomach and activate the stretch receptors without over-consuming calories. Beans and rice or potatoes with a large salad fill the stomach with only 400-500 calories, while filling the stomach with chicken and cheese can take as much as 3400 calories!

In an attempt to reduce calorie consumption, many people make the mistake of trying to eat only fruits and vegetables. While these are incredibly nutritious foods, they are too low in calorie density to be relied on exclusively. A pound of vegetables will fill your stomach, but with only 100 calories or so, the nutrient receptors will detect inadequate calorie intake and you will still feel hungry. This is why fruits and vegetables, while very important, appear a little higher on our pyramid.

This diet is high in carbohydrate, very low in protein and fat, and should include 45 or more grams of fiber per day (people often report that eating this way is a "moving experience!").

These dietary parameters surprise many people, who've been taught that foods like potatoes are fattening. The advice to avoid the consumption of starchy foods is based on erroneous assumptions that these foods are high in calories and that consuming them results in rapid rises in blood sugar levels and increased insulin response. These assumptions are simply not true. Starchy foods are low in calories, high in fiber, and densely nutritious.

The only potential problem with these foods is the way they are prepared. Baked potatoes are commonly topped with sour cream and butter; potatoes are fried and served as French fries; corn on the cob is slathered with butter or olive oil; and beans and rice are accompanied by pork and cheese. It is the added dairy, meat, fat, and oil that make starchy foods fattening, not the foods themselves.

Treats are not part of the daily fare and are therefore at the top of the pyramid. It is important to differentiate between *food* and *treats*. Treats include things such as chocolate, cookies and cake, while foods are things like sweet potatoes, salad, and black bean soup. A major contributing factor to the development of health problems is that the blurring of the distinction between food and treats. Treats are fine, but you cannot treat yourself several times per day and expect to achieve optimal health.

The easiest way to make treats an occasional indulgence is to practice "situational" consumption. For example, have cake at a birthday party, but do not keep cake at your home or office. If you keep cakes, cookies and candies in your house, they will call your name from the kitchen until you finally give in and eat them. Stock your house and office with lots of healthy foods, like soup, wraps, fruits, and vegetables. Make it easier to make the right choices regularly, rather than easy to make the wrong ones.

Why A Plant-Based Diet?

Dr. T. Colin Campbell, Jacob Gould Schurman Professor Emeritus of Nutritional Science at Cornell University, has spent decades researching the connection between diet and health. He conducted the most comprehensive study examining the relationship between nutrition and disease ever undertaken. His findings were remarkable and contradict much of the information still distributed about diet and health today.

Dr. Campbell grew up on a dairy farm and spent his early career researching how to increase protein yields from livestock. An article in an obscure Indian medical journal concluding that animal protein was a cancer promoter caught his attention, and would turn out to be the catalyst that eventually resulted in a complete change in his beliefs about diet.

Dr. Campbell received grants from the National Institutes of Health to explore the relationship between animal protein and cancer with researchers at Cornell. The goal of the research was to replicate the findings of the Indian researchers, and to determine the mechanism of action by which animal protein promoted tumor growth.

Early research was conducted on lab rats, which were given aflatoxin (a known cancer-causing agent) and then fed diets with varying amounts of animal protein.   At the beginning of Dr. Campbell's research, the assumption was that protein intake altered how aflatoxin was detoxified by enzymes in the liver, and research was focused on the effect of protein on enzymes that can both detoxify and activate aflatoxin. The research clearly showed that protein consumption at 5% of total calories greatly decreased the toxicity of aflatoxin and its potential to cause cancer.

Further experiments yielded increasingly interesting results. Foci are clusters of cells that grow into tumors. Dr. Campbell's team measured the effect of protein consumption on the development of foci, and determined that foci development was almost entirely dependent upon how much animal protein was consumed, no matter how much aflatoxin was administered. In fact, when low-protein diets were fed to high-aflatoxin groups, and high protein diets were fed to low-aflatoxin groups, animals fed the high-aflatoxin diet with low protein experienced much lower development of foci than those fed the low-aflatoxin diets with high amounts of protein.   Another astounding development was that when animals experiencing increases in foci activity as a result of a high animal protein diet were converted to a diet of 5%

animal protein, foci development was reduced sharply. When the 20% protein diet was introduced again, foci development increased substantially. In other words, Dr. Campbell and his researchers were turning cancer on and off in the laboratory simply by manipulating the percentage of animal protein in the diet.

By far one of the most important conclusions of this phase of Dr. Campbell's research was that not all proteins had the same cancer-promoting effect. Organic milk protein was used in these experiments. The researchers repeated the experiments with soy and wheat proteins. The results – plant protein did not promote cancer growth even at higher levels of intake. It was clearly animal protein that promoted cancer growth.

Dr. Campbell and his team also evaluated other health measurements in the lab rats. The low protein rats lived longer, were more physically active, were thinner and had healthy hair coats at 100 weeks, while all of the rats fed a high-protein were dead by that time. The low-protein rats also ate more calories and burned more calories than those fed the high-protein diet.

Dr. Campbell's team went on to receive funding to study the effects of nutrition on other carcinogens, such as hepatitis B, and the results were identical – rats with hepatitis B experienced no cancer when consuming 5% of calories from animal protein, while 100% of those consuming 20% of calories from animal protein did.

An important question remained, however - was the experience of the rats relevant to humans? There were reasons to believe that the answer might be "yes." Rats and humans have similar protein needs, and protein is metabolized in rats and humans in similar ways. In both rodents and humans the initiation stage of cancer is far less important than the promotion stage. And, the level of protein intake in the research was proportional to protein intake in humans today.

In the early 1970's the Premier of China was dying from cancer. He directed the government to conduct a survey of death rates for 12 different kinds of cancer in 800 million Chinese citizens. This survey involved 650,000 researchers and was the largest research project undertaken in history. The results were published in a "Cancer Atlas," which showed that cancer rates varied greatly in the different geographic areas of China. This was significant since 98% of the people in China at the time were from the same ethnic group, the Han people.

This caught the interest of Dr. Campbell, particularly when he read another study prepared for the U.S. Congress in 1981 concluding that only 2-3% of cancer risk is based on genes.[28] An obvious potential theory to explore was that diet and environment might be the principle causes of cancer.

The China Study was the first major collaborative research project between the U.S. and China. Data was gathered on 367 variables from adults in 65 counties, through questionnaires, blood tests, and urine samples. Everything families ate was measured for 3 days and food samples from markets around the country were analyzed. By the time the data were gathered, there were over 94,000 correlations identified, 8000 of them statistically significant associations between diet and disease. This is still the largest and most comprehensive study of its type ever undertaken.

Dr. Campbell's team reported that in China, the diet is quite different from ours. Americans take in 15-16% of calories from protein and 80% of this protein is from animal foods. Chinese people eat a diet with 9-10% protein and only 10% of it comes from animal foods.

Chinese people have cholesterol levels ranging from 70-170 mg/dl. In other words, their high is our average, and their low is still considered by many to be dangerously low. Low cholesterol levels were found to be correlated with low rates of not only heart disease, but also other diseases too. As cholesterol levels in Chinese people decreased from 170 mg/dl to 90 mg/dl, there were corresponding lower rates of cancers of the lung, liver, rectum, colon, breast; as well as childhood leukemia, adult leukemia, childhood and adult brain cancer, and stomach and esophageal cancer.

The correlation between low cholesterol levels and low rates of cardiovascular disease is corroborated by the findings of Dr.

William Castelli, former director of the Framingham Study. He reported that in this 50-year project, not one person who maintained a cholesterol level of 150 mg/dl or lower has had a heart attack.[29]

What accounts for high blood cholesterol? The answer might surprise you. *Animal protein* in the diet was the number one link to higher blood cholesterol levels, much more so than dietary cholesterol and fat.

Nonetheless, fat intake was lower in rural China, 14.5% of calories, as compared with about 36% of calories for Americans. Fat consumption increased as animal food consumption increased.

The statistical relationship between animal food intake and cancer rates was true for many forms of cancer. Family cancer rates were directly tied to animal food consumption and this relationship held true even at very low intakes of animal foods.

Fiber consumption was higher in the Chinese people due to their increased intake of plant foods – roughly 3 times the intake of Americans. Some "experts" in the U.S. have preached for years that too much fiber can be dangerous, particularly affecting the absorption of iron. However, there was no sign of iron deficiency in these Chinese people.

Another conclusion from this massive study was the observation that the Chinese consume more calories daily, about 30% more per kg of body weight than Americans. Yet the body weight of these people was an average of 20% lower. It appears that a high-fat, high- protein diet encourages the storage of calories as body fat, since the body is unable to efficiently use the excess for fuel. A diet comprised of foods higher in complex carbohydrates provides energy which is used for higher metabolic function and physical activity. Chinese people consume more calories and maintain lower body weight both because they are more physically active *and* because they consume the right foods.

Chinese eating habits have changed over the last several years, particularly in the major cities. As Chinese people have become wealthier and more Westernized, their diets have become more and more Americanized. An unfortunate byproduct of these changes has been a significant increase in the rates of heart disease, cancer, diabetes, and obesity. In many of the rural areas, Chinese people have continued to eat a traditional diet and the rates of degenerative diseases have remained relatively low.

Should I Eat Animal Foods?

A strong case can be made for eliminating dairy foods from everyone's diet. Cow's milk products have been linked to many conditions, including juvenile diabetes,[30][31][32] multiple sclerosis,[33] chronic ear infections,[34][35] and prostate cancer.[36]

There are no cultures that eat a totally plant-based diet. Some healthy, hardy populations include some animal foods in their diets; however the amounts are quite small as a percentage of calories. But the consumption of animal foods is not required in order to achieve and maintain optimal health. Human nutrition needs can be easily met with a well-structured plant-based diet.

If you do choose to consume animal foods, restrict consumption to small portions only 2-3 times per week, and make sure that the animal foods you do eat are organic (the steroids, hormones and antibiotics administered to conventionally-grown livestock are extremely detrimental to health) or wild-caught if you are eating fish.

There is no question that the fastest and most positive changes in health and weight take place when one eliminates animal foods, and that a totally plant-based diet is the best protection against disease. In fact, there are no nutrients in animal foods which cannot be consumed in plant foods, with the possible exception of vitamin B12. Additionally, the consumption of whole plant foods does not involve the risks associated with the consumption of animal foods.

About The Wellness Forum's Philosophy

Some people are surprised that the Wellness Forum's diet allows for the consumption of some animal foods, and this has generated controversy in some circles.

The Wellness Forum's inclusion of animal foods is accompanied by several qualifiers. Our plan allows for those who are not sick, or are only mildly sick (20 pounds overweight, with no other health concerns, for example) to continue to eat animal foods. The most recent version of our food guide places animal foods toward the top, accompanied by the term "optional," which means that animal foods are not a *necessary* part of the diet or a requirement for optimal health. We instruct that only organic animal foods and wild fish should be consumed; that cow's milk products should be eliminated; and that calories from animal foods should not exceed 10% of overall calories. In other words, our members consume animal foods two to three times per week, while eating plant-based fare the rest of the time.

We strongly recommend that people who are suffering from coronary artery disease, type-2 diabetes, and other serious conditions, convert to a low-fat vegan diet, and we provide ample published scientific evidence showing that doing so gives them the best chance to experience significant health improvement.

There are several reasons why we continue to allow small amounts of organic animal food as part of our main dietary plan for most people. The first is that there is no evidence that a vegan diet is *required* in order for the maintenance of optimal health. In fact, studies of populations with very low disease rates, such as the rural Chinese and northern Africans, have shown that these people do eat small amounts of animal foods. Their eating patterns are based on economics, since plant foods are cheaper and these populations are not generally wealthy, but the fact remains that they are not vegan.

The Wellness Forum's dietary recommendations are based on what the best science shows to be the best diet for humans, not on my personal preferences or habits, or anyone's or any group's political agenda or point of view. We simply cannot back up the statement that a vegan diet is *required* in order for a person in generally good health to remain that way.

One area in which almost everyone agrees (including some of my critics on this issue), is that we must get the message about how diet can affect health outcomes to more people, specifically to more mainstream audiences. I agree, but if we are going to do this, we have to deliver a message that is defensible, and that people are willing to listen to. The Wellness Forum has been incredibly successful precisely because we have reached the "not yet sick" and "mildly sick" with our message, in addition to people who are very sick. Thousands of these types of people have made huge changes in their diet, the most significant of which are the reduction of animal foods and an increase in plant food consumption.

Many if not most of these people would not have even listened if we had started with our most strict dietary recommendations (the ones we reserve for the sickest people). I do not consider it a good outcome to send a 31-year-old person eating some version of the Standard American Diet back into the world to continue doing so until he is really sick and then willing to agree to any form of restriction in order to recover. I want to get that person to start changing his or her habits *before* disaster strikes, and to do so, I must put forth a plausible and defensible plan.

The reality is that many of our clients, once they get started, end up making much more sweeping changes than they originally intended to make. Our files are filled with "accidental vegans" – people who just drifted in that direction and eventually decided that this diet and lifestyle was for them, or became more knowledgeable about issues like factory farming and changed their habits accordingly. We have found that if you can get someone to take a step in the right direction, you can generally get them to take more steps. They key is to get them walking down the path to better health in the first place, an option that does not exist if we scare significant portions of the population off during our initial interaction.

Now, at the risk of offending some people, I'm going to discuss another important point concerning people who do not eat animal foods and think that we should promote a diet free of all animal foods. The reason why people check out organizations like The Wellness Forum is that they are interested in improving their health. Unfortunately, many of the vegans in America are not doing a very good job of modelling health for the rest of the population. It is true that they have eliminated animal foods, but many vegans are still eating a horrible diet with too much fat and the inclusion of lots of processed foods. Many of them are overweight and unhealthy; we deal with this population consistently. I do not recall the last time I attended a vegetarian or vegan event where I did not encounter a significant number of people who were overweight or unhealthy-looking. This certainly does not entice people into wanting to become vegan; in fact it screams to them than that a vegan diet is not a healthy one.

Many of our clients who continue to eat small amounts of animal foods are lean, active, have healthy biomarkers, and they look great. I'll compare these clients with unhealthy vegans (who are, unfortunately, quite common), and they come out ahead every time.

It *is* possible to be a responsible meat eater. It is possible to reduce your carbon foot print significantly by restricting animal foods in the way our general plan prescribes. If we could get all Americans to do this, we would dry up demand for animal foods produced on factory farms, and we would significantly reduce the incidence of heart disease, cancer, and other degenerative conditions. This, in turn, would ratchet down health care costs dramatically since most health care dollars are spent taking care of people suffering from diseases caused by poor diet and lifestyle choices.

I'm starting with the assumption that we all agree that our objectives are to improve public health, reduce health care costs, eliminate factory farms, and reduce the negative environmental impact resulting from our current eating habits. If that's the case, let's agree to meet members of the public where they are and make it attractive for them to join us.

Del's Story

My weight problems started as a child. I remember being put on a diet of only 800 calories per day when I was only eight years old. I overate and my mother dealt with that by forcing me to do portion control. It didn't work; my weight problems carried over into adulthood.

A few years ago, I started my own business, a vegan bakery, and converted to vegan eating at that time. I had previously worked in a "health food" restaurant, which I later learned, was not so healthy after all. That is where my consumption of vegan junk food really began.

Believe it or not, I gained 100 pounds within one year, and the weight gain continued until I peaked out at 460 pounds! You might be wondering how an individual consuming a vegan diet could accomplish this. Here's how I did it.

Every day, I started my day with two fresh scones and coffee. Then, I proceeded to eat a cashew bar and muffin for lunch, or cake or whatever was handy – I was working very hard and rarely sat down to eat a full meal. I continued to munch on sugary foods and drink caffeine-filled beverages throughout the day and for "real meals" I would eat vegetarian foods prepared with lots of oil and fat. In the evenings to relax, I'd eat potato chips and drink beer. All vegan, but certainly not healthy!

In summer of 2005, I reached my wit's end. I was exhausted. My body ached, my knees ached. I fell and my injured ankle would not heal. I needed help!

I went to my good friend Dr. Pam Popper and told her I was ready to change my life! I immediately converted to a well-structured plant-based diet; instead of scones and coffee for breakfast I started having fruit smoothies and whole grain cereal. I replaced my constant snacking with meals comprised of beans, whole grains, potatoes and salads. And, the weight started coming off right away.

It was not easy – I craved some of the bad foods for a long time, and was very tempted to resume my old eating patterns, since they were familiar to me, particularly when I was stressed. Although I did cheat once in a while, the thing that kept me from reverting back was being accountable to Dr. Pam, and the desire to get this problem behind me once and for all!

I lost 50 pounds in the first six months, and hit a plateau, at which time Dr. Pam told me I had to start moving. I started walking, since that was the least painful thing I could do. The weight started dropping again.

At 75 pounds, I hit another plateau, and the advice was to step up the exercise. This is when I started working out with Dr. Pam and taking Wellness Forum Hot Yoga classes. And that is when the weight started dropping like crazy. People started telling me I looked different almost from day to day. I must confess that stepping up the exercise program was the most miserable thing I have ever done in my life. I used to hiss at Dr. Pam in the gym, and lay on my yoga mat praying for death. Fortunately this did not last long, and although I hated to admit it, I started to enjoy getting in shape. I actually missed working out when my schedule caused me to miss a day.

I still have another 50 pounds to lose, but it's getting easier and easier every day. I don't even have to think about things most days. I just eat the way I've formed the habit of eating, do the required exercise, and the weight comes off.

Here's the best part – I am working harder than I have ever worked in my life, and I am less tired as a result of doing it. My ankle is finally healing (I hated the calf raises for weeks, but they do work!). I am wearing clothes that I haven't worn for years. I feel great about myself. I may even run a marathon with Dr. Pam since I have all of this energy now.

So, let me emphasize a couple of things. First, conversion to a vegan diet does not, in and of itself, lead to health. You have to convert to a *well-structured* vegan diet. I have quit sabotaging myself – the wrong foods are like drugs for me and when I think about not eating healthfully, I remember my goals and I don't eat them. I am learning to make self-care a priority – no matter how busy I am, I make time to eat good food and to exercise. And I try to be around like-minded people who reinforce my good habits.

Feeling good feels good and I have no desire to return to the way I used to be.

Knowing vs. Doing

It is much easier for people to understand the diet and lifestyle changes they need to make than it is to actually make the changes. In other words knowing what to do does not necessarily translate into doing the right things. Why? The reasons range from simple lack of discipline to emotional problems that cause people to overeat.

I know my limitations – I'm not a therapist and I refer people who need therapy to good people who are specialists in this area. But I am really good at time management, communicating simple strategies for making changes, and teaching people how to set themselves up for success.

As the authors of *Influencer* state in the above quote, you have organized yourself in a way that promotes certain behaviors, some of which affect your health outcomes. In all likelihood, you did this without much conscious thought. If you want to develop different behaviors that lead to better outcomes, you will need to deliberately make some changes in the way you organize your day-to-day life. Below are some of the strategies I use to keep myself on track;
none of them are particularly original, but they are effective.

Sanitize your environment. You've heard this before, but you *must* get the forbidden foods out of your house and office, and anyplace else you spend time. This cleansing has to include all of the healthier junk foods too – the baked chips, fruit juice-sweetened cookies, and soy ice cream. Many of you are still trying to discipline yourself to choose between apples and ice cream and sooner or later ice cream will win. Make it easy to make the right choices and harder to make wrong choices.

Plan ahead. You have to make time to shop for food, and to do some basic preparation in order to have healthy foods ready to eat. I always have cooked rice, frozen vegetables, oats, plant milk, smoothie mix, fruit, pre-washed greens, canned beans, instant soups, and other such foods handy. If I'm in a hurry, a bag of frozen vegetables with some brown rice is a great quick lunch or dinner. Not a gourmet feast, but basic food that is filling and tasty. Chopped romaine lettuce, tomatoes, cucumbers and fat-free dressing taste great; steamed kale with marinara sauce; leftover soup with added rice; black bean and rice burritos; and vegetable wraps; these are all quick foods that will keep you from reaching for unhealthy convenience foods you should not eat. Get organized and set your kitchen up to promote health!

Tell everyone you spend time with that you have changed your diet. While there is a risk that you may hear some lectures about being protein deficient or other such nonsense, telling others about your new diet and lifestyle will increase the odds that you will stay on the straight and narrow path when you're around these people. It's hard to tell people that you're going to eat a low-fat plant-based diet and then order cheese pizza for dinner and brownies for dessert.

Stop making excuses. Humans are very good at justifying their choices and behavior – I can be very skilled at this myself. But at some point you have to stop giving reasons for not doing what you're supposed to do and just do what you know is right. Easier said than done, but once you get in the habit, life becomes easier overall.

Schedule your exercise sessions and stick with your schedule. I realized some time ago that most people do not have a good scheduling method that insures time to work out and to fit in other important activities too. So here's some detail on how I arrange my schedule that really works for me. It's a method called default scheduling and it will not only allow you to fit everything in, but help you to do so without much stress.

I use an appointment book called Quo Vadis Trinote which I purchase from the Daily Planner. I am an old fashioned girl who needs to see an entire week at a time in order to make best use of my time, and seeing it on paper works best for me. I get my appointment book in early Oct for the next year and the first thing I do is write in all of the recurring things I do – my monthly CEO group, my book club, trips and speaking engagements, birthdays and other dates to remember, etc. This is done by mid-October.

I set my schedule a few weeks in advance – when I'm going to do on-on-one appointments (I block off times for the staff to fill in), when we will have staff meetings, and other such important activities. There's lots of detail in terms of how I organize things like to-do lists and projects that we don't need to cover here (perhaps some time I'll schedule a time management conference call to provide more detail!).

At the beginning of each week I schedule in workouts, runs, and yoga classes for the following week and *write them down in my book*. In other words, I don't get up every morning and hope I'll find the time to exercise – I know a week in advance not only *when* I'll be exercising but exactly *what* I'll be doing during those allotted times. I don't allow anything (other than death and sickness – my own) to stand in the way of those appointments – I schedule around them. It is not unusual to get 3-4 requests to do something, call someone, or be available for each exercise time I have scheduled. I generally respond and agree to those requests, but insist that they be scheduled at a time that does not interfere with my scheduled exercise sessions. I would never miss a plane because someone wanted me to talk to a prospect when I'm scheduled to leave for the airport; I do not miss workouts for those reasons either.

Do it whether you feel like it or not. Don't give in to yourself. Ever. Well almost not ever; sometimes things do happen like ice storms or serious illness. But on a day-to-day basis, people tell me they missed yoga classes and workouts because they had a headache, did not sleep well last night, pulled a muscle, had a huge project due, and many other such reasons. Stop this. It is a great way to undermine your plans to be fit and healthy. And, I've found that the way people approach exercise is often the way they approach other things too, like work. Get in the habit of doing the things you are supposed to when you've agreed to do them, regardless of whether or not it's convenient, or you want to or really feel like doing them. You'll be a better employee or business owner; a better parent; a better member of your community; and a better person.

Stop telling yourself stories; that you don't have time, this new plan won't work, your kids need something that keeps you from eating well and exercising, and other negative self-talk. My definition of negative self-talk is any conversation you have either with yourself or others that promotes the idea that you cannot change your circumstances. Stop looking for reasons why this won't work and start figuring out how to make it work. Both involve about the same amount of energy; but the results are entirely different.

Remember that the things that seem the most restrictive are the things that set you free. Some people look at my life, which is scheduled and planned and includes lots of exercise and foods like steamed kale and think that my life must be really limited. The opposite is true. Because I am organized, and I schedule and plan, I have time to do all the things I'm supposed to do (work, diet, exercise) and time to other things too - belong to a book club, read, activities with friends, shop, travel, go to movies, play with my cat, spend time with my family and other things that are important. The restrictions I place on myself provide me the freedom to do the things I want to do. And the best part is I have great health and lots of energy so I can enjoy all of these things!

So get started now! This is really it. You're either going to do it or not. If you really want to change your life, you can. Today. Now. Right now. Ok that's all because I'm going to yoga class.

Myths and Misunderstandings

It's Not Your Genes!
Fats and Oils
Protein
Supplements
Confusing Information

It's Not Your Genes, It's Your Diet!

By far the most hopeful information that people learn in my lectures and in Wellness Forum classes is that genes are not the principal determinant of health. If you go through life thinking that your health is based on your genes, you are essentially a helpless victim. On the other hand, once you understand that your *choices* determine your health outcomes, you're in control!

Research shows that having certain genes may indeed predispose you to develop conditions like cancer, diabetes, and obesity. But how those genes express themselves is largely based on the way you live your life; your diet and lifestyle choices. Genes can remain dormant, or they can be "switched on" by the way you live your life, most importantly, the foods that you eat.

This is not to say that genes are not important. They are. They are important for every human function. But there is very convincing evidence that your health status is predominantly influenced by what you put in your mouth every day, much more so than by your genes.

Obesity and disease rates in the U.S. have increased significantly in the last several decades; the obesity rate more than doubled between 1980 and 2000,[37] the diabetes rate doubled in only ten years between 1997 and 2007,[38] and the number of deaths from heart disease doubled between 1940 and 2000.[39] The genetic code of human beings could not have changed enough during this period of time in order to explain the rapid increases in the incidence of these diseases.

The increased rate of disease is a result of changes in dietary patterns during the last several decades. Calorie consumption increased from 2,234 calories per person per day in 1970 to 2757 calories per day in 2003. Between 1970 and 2003, per capita consumption of fats and oils increased by 63%, and sugars and sweeteners by 19%. The consumption of corn sweeteners alone increased by 400% between 1970 and 2003.[40]

Lessons From The Pima Indians

The Pima Indians provide a great opportunity to compare the effects of diet vs. genes on the development of certain diseases. There are two major communities of Pima Indians; one group lives in the Sierra Madre Mountains in Mexico and the other group lives in Arizona.

The two groups are descendants from the same families; many married within their own community; and multiple generations of families live in the same area, allowing researchers to track changes in the habits and the disease rates of both groups. Millions of dollars have been invested in researching these people by the National Institutes of Health.

Most of the Mexican Pima Indians are physically active, either because they are engaged in farming or because they have jobs involving manual labor. For example, women spend an average of 22 hours per week engaged in some form of physical activity, much of which is quite demanding. The Mexican Pima eat a diet that is low in fat and high in fiber, with the average Pima consuming more than 50 grams of fiber per day.

The Arizona Pima Indians enjoy a very Americanized lifestyle, including the consumption of a diet high in animal protein and fat. These Indians are far less active than their Mexican counterparts; women spend only 3.1 hours per week engaged in any form of physical activity.

The differences in diet and lifestyle are reflected in differences in the health status of these groups, particularly in the incidence of diabetes. 6.9% of the Pima Indians living in Mexico have diabetes, as compared to 38% of the Arizona Pima .[41]

Almost all studies involving these communities have concluded that diet is responsible for the differences in health outcomes between the two groups. One research group wrote, "The much lower prevalence of type 2 diabetes and obesity in the Pima Indians in Mexico than in the U.S. indicates that even in populations genetically prone to these conditions, their development is determined mostly by environmental circumstances, thereby suggesting that type 2 diabetes is largely preventable. This study provides compelling evidence that changes in lifestyle associated with Westernization play a major role in the global epidemic of type 2 diabetes.[42]

Genes and Cancer

Incredible sums of money have been invested in studying the human genome, looking for the genetic origin of disease. In 1994, mutations to the BRCA-1 and BRCA-2 genes, predisposing women to develop breast cancer, were discovered.

But breast cancer cannot be attributed solely to genetic predisposition. Only one in five hundred women carry the mutated versions of these genes,[43] yet the American Cancer Society states that one in eight American women will develop breast cancer in her lifetime.[44] In other words, not all women who carry the gene mutation develop breast cancer, and many women who are do not have these mutated genes do. In fact, according to one study, less than 3% of all breast cancers are attributable to genes.[45]

So if genes are not the predictor of who will get breast cancer, what is? Diet!

Migration Studies

Many studies have shown that when people move from one area to another and start eating the typical diet of their new home, they soon have the same disease risk of the area to which they moved.[46]

For example, Japanese women in the U.S. are significantly more likely to develop breast cancer than Japanese women living in Japan and other Asian countries.[47] One of the reasons is that the traditional Japanese diet is lower in fat, particularly saturated animal fat, than the typical Westernized diet. In the 1940's breast cancer was relatively rare in Japan, and at that time the Japanese diet was comprised of less than 10% of calories from fat.[48]

But within a short time after moving to the U.S., Japanese women have the same risk of breast cancer as American women.

Their genetic makeup does not change as they fly across the ocean to their new homes; the main cause is the increase in consumption of fat, particularly fat in animal foods.

The same holds true for other populations and other conditions. Disease rates tend to be related to diet and lifestyle habits, rather than attributable to ethnicity.

Dr. Jane Powley's Story

When I was growing up in China, 99.9% of our diet was plant-based food. This was not because we read *The China Study*; it was the traditional diet. It was inexpensive and my family did not have a lot of money. We didn't have a refrigerator in my home, so we went to the market to purchase rice, beans, fruit, and vegetables almost every day. At that time, almost 60 years ago, the government issued permits that allowed families to get eight ounces of cooking oil and about two ounces of meat per person each month. Even people with money could not get more because these foods were rationed. We used those foods very sparingly because they were scarce. For special occasions, like the Chinese New Year, we would get coupons for white flour and white rice.

I came to the U.S. to attend graduate school at the University of Maryland. When I arrived, I weighed about 130 pounds and I was eating a traditional Chinese diet of rice, vegetables and beans. I shared an office with another graduate student, and one day she was eating something that smelled so good. I asked her what it was and she told me it was fried chicken. She told me I could buy it at a fast food restaurant in the student center, and since my English was not very good, my new friend instructed me to ask for" two pieces of dark meat chicken." The next day I bought my first dark meat fried chicken. It was delicious!

After a few days, I started noticing that I became tired after lunch so my new friend suggested drinking Coca-Cola with my chicken. It worked! I loved the chicken *and* I had lots of energy. Gradually I found out about other delicious American foods, including ice cream, which I also added to my daily diet.

I really did not understand that there would be health consequences from eating these new foods. I never worried about my weight in China, but soon I needed new clothes because I was gaining weight on my new American diet. I also became more tired and so I started drinking more Coke to get me through the day. Soon other problems, much more serious ones, developed – I had an irregular heartbeat, chronic infections, pneumonia, digestive problems, an ulcer, and many other health issues.

I transferred to the University of Delaware and during the very first semester I was hospitalized. Shortly after, I met my future husband, Dr. Chuck Powley. By this time, I weighed 188 pounds and my health problems had progressed. I'm lucky because Chuck loved me even though I was at my heaviest and sickest. He told me not to worry because we had great insurance, and he sent me to doctors who gave me prescription drugs. My condition continued to get worse, so I consulted a Chinese herbalist. I still did not get better and I was still gaining weight; I know now that it was because I was still eating the American diet.

When things were about as bad as they could be, someone gave me a tape of a lecture by Dr. Pam Popper and it really made an impression on me. I flew to Columbus and learned about the plant-based diet. I made the decision to adopt it right away, flew home and started eating only plant foods. I went back to the peasant-style diet I ate as a child in China.

My husband encouraged me because he understood that this new diet could make me well, but he did not want to eat this way. For a while, he ate dinner out; he said he didn't want to eat "Jane food."

Gradually, the weight fell off, I stopped taking all the medications, and my health issues resolved. I have not even taken an over-the-counter drug since 1994! I was so excited that I opened a center in Wilmington, Delaware, to offer the classes developed by Dr. Pam. Now I help other people change their health and their lives like Dr. Pam helped me!

Over time, I learned to make "Jane food" more delicious, and eventually Chuck asked if he could join me at the dinner table again. Since then, he has also learned to cook tasty "Jane food" – in fact he attended cooking classes at my center to learn how to make healthy, delicious foods for me!

Today, when I go home to China, I see more and more Chinese people, especially the younger generation, eating an American diet. Fast food restaurants are everywhere, the government no longer regulates the availability of meats and oils, and people with money can afford to eat foods that destroy health. Heart disease, cancer and diabetes are all increasing in the major cities. It breaks my heart to see this.

I love my new diet and lifestyle, I love being healthy, and I love helping others. Clients ask me for advice and I tell them the most important thing to remember is that little changes do not work. You have to change the whole diet in order to get results. They ask how long you have to commit to this lifestyle and I tell them it is for the rest of your life – and then I tell them they will be rewarded for the rest of their lives too!

Identical Twins

Some of the most convincing studies about the influence of diet vs. genes have been done on identical twins. Identical twins have almost identical DNA. However, they generally live separately as adults, and often their diets and lifestyle habits develop quite differently. Studies of identical twins provide great opportunities to look at how differing diets can result in differing health outcomes.

One study showed that among identical twins, that when one twin developed type-2 diabetes, the other twin had less than a 40% chance of developing it. The differences in outcomes were attributed to environmental factors, particularly diet.[49]

Researchers at The University of Michigan looked at 11 pairs of identical twins, in which one twin in each pair had rheumatoid arthritis. There are genes that predispose people to develop RA, but only 15% of identical twins will both develop it. The researchers concluded that non-genetic factors (like diet) explained how two people who are so biologically alike could experience such different health outcomes.[50]

The Bottom Line

During the last 15 years, we have helped thousands of people to regain their health using plant-based nutrition. Many of these people came from families in which many people had diabetes, cancer, or heart disease. The principle determining factor as to whether or not clients will get better has never been family history; it has always willingness to adopt and maintain a well-structured plant-based diet.

Fats and Oils

As you probably have gathered from what you have already read, there is much "common knowledge" about nutrition that is incorrect based on the published scientific literature. But these misunderstandings and misinterpretations of the data are continually perpetuated by nutrition and health professionals, magazines, books and television shows. This is certainly the case with fats and oils.

Misinformation has convinced people that consuming so-called "good fats" allows for the consumption of *more* fat, and that the *type* of fat is more important than the *amount* of fat. Many people even think that they *must* consume certain fats, like olive oil, in order to enjoy optimal health. Most people are absolutely *astounded* when I say that olive oil is not a health food in my lectures.

How did the myths about oils and fats get started and why are they still being told? Part of the answer is that research is often misreported, and some very good studies are not reported at all. Many doctors have little nutrition training, and most do not spend much time researching diet-related issues. Lack of training often results in the acceptance of statements made about nutrition in books and at conferences without further investigation to confirm or refute the information they learn. These doctors, and often other health care professionals too, then tell their patients to do many incorrect things, such as consuming foods like olive oil and fish. Since most people think that foods that contain fat taste good, advice to eat them from supposedly learned nutrition professionals and doctors is well-received.

The promotion of the health benefits of olive oil really started in the 1950's when an American nutritionist, Ansel Keys, discovered that men living on the island of Crete had very low rates of heart disease and cancer and seemed to be experiencing longer life spans. Intrigued, he conducted a 15-year study in which heart disease and cancer rates were studied in Greece (Crete and Corfu), Finland, Japan, Italy, the Netherlands, the United States, and Yugoslavia. This was known as the "Seven-

Country Study," and it showed that in Crete and Japan, the rates of heart disease were lower than in the other five countries.[51]

It was true that residents of Crete consumed olive oil – about three tablespoons per day. But they also practiced many healthy habits – they consumed lots of fruits, vegetables and whole grains, and their physical activity levels were very high – the equivalent of nine miles of walking per day (most residents were engaged in some form of agriculture at that time). Their health status certainly could not be attributed to the consumption of olive oil alone, and one could argue that the other healthy habits practiced by these people helped to overcome what we now know are the detrimental effects of regularly consuming oils of any type.

Today, the residents of Crete continue to consume olive oil. But their meat and fish intake has increased in recent years, and as a result their health status has declined.[52] Sixty percent of adults and 50% of children are overweight, and the rates of heart disease, cancer and diabetes have increased dramatically.[53] But the decline in the health status of these people is not limited to the consumption of animal foods only. One relatively recent study of people living on the island of Crete determined that patients *with* heart disease consumed more monounsaturated fat daily than patients *without* heart disease. The more olive oil consumed, the more heart disease they developed.[54]

The idea that olive oil is a health food really became popular when some of the findings of the Lyon Diet Heart Study were made public. In this study, French researchers divided 605 participants into two groups, one of which consumed a Mediterranean-style diet that:

- was high in fruits, vegetables, bread, cereals, beans, nuts and seeds
- contained olive oil as a source of monounsaturated fat
- included dairy products, fish and poultry with little red meat
- called for eggs 2-4 times per week
- allowed wine in moderate amounts

The other group was given no dietary advice, but was advised by physicians to eat a diet described by the American Heart Association as "comparable to what is typically consumed in the United States."

Those on the experimental diet were between 50% and 70% less likely to experience adverse cardiovascular events and death than those consuming some version of the Standard American Diet. The media immediately started promoting the health benefits of the Mediterranean Diet, with particular focus on red wine and olive oil. The 50-70% reduction in the rate of heart disease was impressive, and these results should not be entirely discounted.

But all of the findings from this study were not well-publicized. By the end of the study, 25% of the participants consuming the Mediterranean Diet had experienced a cardiovascular event or had died. Again, these results were better than those experienced eating a traditional American diet,[55] but we now know, based on results from The China Study and the work of Dr. Caldwell Esselstyn, that the rates of heart disease can be ratcheted down even further by consuming a low-fat, plant-based diet.

Unfortunately, the misunderstandings about fat do not end with olive oil.

Fat Basics and Essential Fatty Acids

There are three basic categories of fats; saturated, polyunsaturated, and monounsaturated. Unsaturated fats are usually in the form of oils, and saturated fats are found in solid animal fats. All fat in foods, however, contains combinations of saturated, polyunsaturated, and monounsaturated fats; the most concentrated form of fat determines how the food is categorized.

There are two *essential* fatty acids, called such because the body is unable to produce them; therefore they must be consumed in foods. These are linolenic acid and linoleic acid. They are used to synthesize other fatty acids, to build cell membranes; for the production of hormones, and for energy metabolism.

A series of biochemical processes allows the body to take linolenic and linoleic acids and convert them to other fatty acids such as:

Gamma-linolenic acid (GLA)
Dihomo-gamma-linoleic acid (DHGLA)
Alpha linolenic acid (ALA)
Eicosapentaenoic acid (EPA)
Docosahexanioc acid (DHA)

Alpha-linolenic acid is the principal precursor to EPA and DHA, which are considered forms of Omega-3 fatty acids and are essential for brain and other important functions.

There is a great deal of confusion about DHA and EPA. These fats *are* important; EPA and DHA are concentrated in brain cells, synapses, retinas, adrenal glands and sex glands. Good dietary sources are fish, eggs, and some sea vegetables, but since the fat content of sea vegetables is very low, these should not be considered a good source. Many health care professionals recommend regular consumption of eggs, fish, or supplementation with fish oil, or DHA and EPA supplements in order to assure adequate intake.

But this is not necessary. EPA and DHA are both made by the body from the alpha-linolenic acid consumed in foods. This is why EPA and DHA are not classified as *essential* fatty acids, while alpha-linolenic acid is. Flax seeds, soy foods and walnuts are good sources of alpha-linolenic acid.

Health care professionals argue that the body does not efficiently convert alpha-linolenic acid to DHA and EPA, necessitating the intake of fish, fish oil, or supplements. It is true that people consuming a poor diet may have difficulty converting essential fatty acids to other long-chain fatty acids. The consumption of trans-fat, excess consumption of saturated fat, and too much intake of Omega-6 fats from land animals and polyunsaturated vegetable oils can interfere with this conversion. However, there is little scientific evidence showing that people consuming a poor diet benefit from the use of supplements in an effort to make up for their dietary indiscretions.

It is true that vegans and vegetarians generally have lower levels of DHA when tested. However, there is no evidence that these lower levels increase the risk of disease, or that supplementation improves health outcomes for these individuals.

Is Fish a Health Food?

Fish such as mackerel, lake trout, herring, sardines, albacore tuna, and salmon are sources of DHA and EPA. However, the benefits of consuming fish have been over-stated. One study that tracked the diets and prostate cancer diagnoses of 18,115 Japanese men concluded that the amount of fish intake was the most significant dietary factor associated with increased risk of prostate cancer. The men who ate fish four or more times per week had a 54% increase in the risk of developing prostate cancer as compared to men who consumed fish fewer than twice a week.[56]

In another study, Finnish researchers concluded that mercury levels associated with fish intake significantly increased the risk of heart disease. Study participants with the highest mercury levels had a 68% increased risk of an acute coronary event and a 68% increased risk for cardiovascular disease in general. Mercury levels were directly related to the amount of fish consumed.[57]

Fish Oils and Omega-3 Supplements

Fish oils are often recommended by doctors and nutrition professionals because of their high DHA and EPA content. The evidence I have reviewed indicates that all oils, including fish oil, are best left out of the diet.

But there are particular concerns with fish oil, including oxidation and rancidity. Dr. Carlene McLean is an oils expert at the New Zealand Crop and Food Research Institute. Dr. McLean says that she has tested fish oil samples from the UK and Asian markets and found that they contain oxidation byproducts, even when evaluated before the sell-by date. The consumption of oxidized oils can increase the risk of heart disease, cancer, and other degenerative conditions.

Studies on the effects of omega-3 supplementation have failed to show improved health outcomes. A study reported in the *British Medical Journal* in April 2006[58] looked at the effects of long and shorter-chain omega-3 fatty acid supplementation on total mortality, cardiovascular events, and cancer. This was a massive study that involved several different research groups and tens of thousands of participants.

The researchers concluded that there was no significant evidence of reduced risk of total mortality or cardiovascular events in participants taking supplemental omega 3 fats. There was a non-significant increase in cancer risk with a higher intake of omega-3, but the researchers could not entirely rule out an increased risk of cancer.

There just is not enough evidence that taking Omega-3 supplements or fish oil improves health outcomes, and perhaps just as important, there is no long-term data evaluating the safety of these products.

Eliminate Oils!

Oils are sources of concentrated fat and calories - one tablespoon of any type of oil has 130 calories and 14 grams of fat. The addition of oils and added fats to the diet make it difficult, if not impossible, for most people to maintain optimal weight and body composition. Just add an oil-based salad dressing to your diet once a day without either decreasing your current calorie intake or increasing the amount of your daily exercise and it is easy to gain 36 pounds in a year!

> 3 Tablespoons of olive oil once per day =
> 3600 extra calories every 10 days;
> this results in weight gain of 3 pounds per month
> or 36 pounds in a year!

Aren't Oils Supposed to be Heart Healthy?

Some oils have been promoted as being heart-healthy, but research shows the opposite to be true.

Dr. David Blankenhorn at the University of Southern California School of Medicine conducted a study in which he compared baseline angiograms with one-year follow-up angiograms in patients with coronary artery disease. Disease progressed just as much for those eating a diet concentrated in monounsaturated fat as those eating saturated fat.[59]

Lawrence Rudel of Wake Forest University conducted experiments feeding varying diets to African Green Monkeys. At the end of five years, monkeys consuming monounsaturated fat had higher HDL and lower LDL levels. But autopsies showed that these monkeys had developed as much coronary disease as those monkeys eating saturated fat. This study not only showed that monounsaturated fats are not healthier, but also that raising HDL levels has little effect on health outcomes, a finding that has also proven true in human studies.[60]

Robert Vogel at the University of Maryland found that consuming bread dipped in olive oil reduced dilation in the brachial artery, indicating injury to the endothelial cells that line the blood vessels and impairment of nitric oxide production.[61] Nitric oxide is a vasodilator, keeping blood vessels open and allowing for efficient blood flow.

Dietary polyunsaturated fats, both omega-3 and omega-6, contribute to the development of human atherosclerotic plaques, damaging the arteries and the contributing to progression of atherosclerosis.[62][63] Most people think that atherosclerotic plaques are made up of saturated fat only.

Research has even shown that consuming oils can cause considerable increases in plasma triglycerides and blood coagulation factors which can lead to a blood clot, which in turn can cause a heart attack or stroke.

In one study, eighteen healthy young men were observed for six consecutive days. One group consumed meals that were fortified with 70 grams of rapeseed oil, olive oil, sunflower oil, palm oil, or butter (42% of calories from fat); the other consumed low-fat meals with about 6% of calories from fat.

Not surprisingly, high-fat meals caused rises in plasma triglycerides, Factor VII (a clotting factor predictive of heart attack risk) and free fatty acids; these effects were not noted after lower-fat meals were consumed. According to the authors, "These findings indicate that high-fat meals may be prothrombotic (causing a blood clot leading to a heart attack), *irrespective of their fatty acid composition* (emphasis mine).[64]

Isn't Fat Needed in order to Absorb Carotenoids and Other Nutrients from Foods?

Although there is scientific evidence that consuming oil-based dressings or higher-fat foods with foods that contain carotenoids increases absorption of them, there is no evidence that this makes a difference in nutrient status or health outcomes. In fact, the evidence is to the contrary; oils and fats contribute to higher risk for degenerative conditions like coronary artery disease, cancer, and diabetes, and more rapid progression of those conditions in spite of the extra absorption of carotenoids.

Furthermore, I am not aware of any degenerative disease that is linked to developing a "carotenoid deficiency," making the consumption of fats and oils as a means to absorb more carotenoids inadvisable and unnecessary.
Another consideration is that low-fat diets reduce oxidative stress, which decreases the need for antioxidants like carotenoids.

Basic Rules for Fat Consumption

After the age of two, human needs for fat are quite low, and should not exceed 15% of total calories for a healthy person. For those individuals who are overweight, or suffering from conditions like coronary artery disease or diabetes, fat consumption should be even lower, at 9-11% of calories.

It's better to consume very small amounts of foods that have a higher fat content (like nuts and seeds), rather than consuming fat that is isolated from foods, like oils. This means ALL oils, not just some oils. This includes olive oil, coconut oil, flax oil, Udo's oil, soybean oil, cottonseed oil, palm oil, peanut oil, fish oil, and just to make sure I cover all the bases – even motor oil!!

Another easy way to reduce fat intake is to significantly reduce or eliminate animal foods from the diet. Even lean animal foods have a very high concentration of fat:

- One 3.5 ounce hamburger made from extra lean ground beef contains 166 calories and 10.28 grams of fat. This equates to 56% of calories from fat!
- 3.5 ounces of lean pork contains 210 calories and 9.58 fat grams – 41% of calories from fat[65]

Learn to prepare foods without the use of oil. For example, stir-fry dishes can be easily prepared using water instead of oil:

Heat your pan over a medium high flame. Add vegetables first, then cook until they start to stick to the pan, tossing gently. Add water, one to two tablespoons at a time to prevent sticking. Do not add too much water as it will steam the vegetables instead of sautéing them.

This sauté method works really well when starting with vegetables like onions, carrots, celery, and peppers, which have a lot of water in them. Other vegetables, like mushrooms, can be added later in the cooking process.

Learn to make fat-free dressings for salads. Oil-based salad dressings are some of the most common hidden sources of fat in the diet. Using enough of an oil-based dressing to flavor a large salad can add as much as 350-500 calories to the dish!

On the next page is an easy and very tasty recipe to get you started:

Orange Dressing by Del Sroufe

This dressing has a very mellow flavor that allows the flavor of the greens to shine. Toss your salad with some fresh orange segments and shaved fennel for a simple but great tasting salad. The agave nectar or brown rice syrup gives the dressing a thickness allowing it to "hold onto" your salad greens.

Ingredients
1/2 cup freshly squeezed orange juice
Zest of 1 orange
4 Tablespoons rice wine vinegar
1/2 cup agave nectar or brown rice syrup
Pinch cayenne pepper—optional
1/4 teaspoon sea salt (optional)

Directions
Combine all ingredients in a medium bowl, and whisk well to combine. Store in an airtight container.
Makes one cup

Learn to use herbs and spices, which add great flavor (much better than oil!); invest in or borrow some good vegetarian cookbooks, and start experimenting.

Non-stick cookware is the best option for low-fat cooking. Instead of using oil to avoid sticking, line baking pans with parchment paper.

Applesauce and bananas are substitutes for oil in baked goods. Pureed prunes or organic baby foods are also great choices. Your baked goods will be much lower in fat and actually taste better too!

When ordering in restaurants, specify that you do not want your vegetables basted in oil or butter, and you want your vegetables steamed rather than stir-fried.

You will not miss the taste of oil! And, your body will not miss all the fat and calories either! Once you stop consuming it for a while, you won't want it, and eating oil-laden foods may even cause intestinal discomfort.

But Where Will I Get My Protein?

Perhaps the most common question asked about plant-based nutrition is "Where do you get your protein?" Protein *is* very important. We absolutely need it, but its significance has been tremendously overstated almost since its discovery in 1839 by Dutch chemist Gerhard Mulder.

There is some justification for concern about protein intake in poor countries, but in industrialized nations where daily calorie intake is adequate, protein needs are easily met.

There are hundreds of thousands of different proteins. The structural and functional components of cells are made of proteins, and protein is a primary component of muscles, hair, skin, and internal organs. Proteins are an important component of our immune systems; they form antibodies to fight bacteria and other foreign invaders. Hemoglobin, which carries oxygen throughout the body, is a protein; so are enzymes, which are catalysts for the body's functions. Hormones such as insulin and estrogen are also proteins. Proteins are built from long chains of hundreds or even thousands of amino acids. Proteins in the body must be replaced regularly, and this is accomplished by eating foods that contain protein.

There are 20 naturally occurring amino acids that comprise proteins. Eight of them are "essential" which means they must be consumed in food; the body can synthesize the others.

Digestion of protein begins in the stomach with exposure to pepsin (an enzyme) which is secreted from digestive juices and activated by hydrochloric acid. Other proteolytic enzymes (those that help with the digestion of protein) are secreted by the pancreas and mucosal cells of the small intestine.

During the process of digestion, proteins from food are broken down into amino acids, which are then absorbed through the small intestine into the bloodstream. These amino acids are then reconstructed to build antibodies, hormones, enzymes, and other cells in the body.

Plant foods contain ample amounts of protein, but most do not contain all eight essential amino acids, which has caused many nutrition experts to label them as inferior sources of protein. The proteins found in plants are often referred to as "incomplete proteins."

Many people, including nutrition professionals, believe that all eight essential amino acids must be consumed at the same time, and that consuming a near-vegetarian or vegan diet requires food to be consumed in specific combinations in order to accomplish this, a concept called "protein complementing."

This theory really became popular when it was mentioned in Frances Moore Lappe's book *Diet for a Small Planet,* published in 1971. Later, scientific evidence showed that it was not necessary to consume all of the essential amino acids at each meal as previously believed. In a later edition of the book published in 1981, Lappe recanted her statements about complementary proteins, but this widely held belief persists to this day.

How Much Protein Do We Really Need?

A unique constituent of protein is nitrogen (carbohydrates and fats do not contain nitrogen). One way to determine how much protein humans need to consume is to measure the amount of nitrogen excreted in the feces, urine, sweat, hair, semen, menstrual fluid, and breath.

Excretion studies have shown that protein needs for normal adults may be as low as 2.5% of calories.[66] This should actually not be surprising; the best food for human babies is human breast milk, which contains only 6% protein,[67] which fuels the most rapid growth humans ever experience.

For over 100 years, researchers have been cautioning that protein needs have been over-stated. In 1905, Russell Henry Chittenden, a Yale Chemistry Professor, published a book called *Physiological Economy in Nutrition,* in which he stated clearly that excess protein consumption was harmful to human health due to toxic byproducts of nitrogen, which are excreted by the kidneys.[68]

Chittenden was not the only scientist who thought that protein needs were much lower than Americans were being advised, but those who were promoting higher protein consumption were a much more vocal and powerful group.

Healthier populations in Asia and Northern Africa consume considerably lower protein diets than Americans, and most of the protein comes from plant foods. All natural foods contain varying amounts of protein, and it is almost impossible to develop a protein deficiency while consuming a varied, whole-foods, plant-based diet that provides adequate daily calories.

The protein content of plants compares well with the protein content of animal foods:[69]

Black Beans	26%
Oatmeal	14.5%
Asparagus	51%
Spinach	57%
Broccoli	42%
Cheddar Cheese	25%
Hamburger	37%
Skim milk	37%
Egg	34%

What Are the Effects of Consuming Too Much Protein?

When you consume protein, it is broken down into amino acids, which are made up of carbon, oxygen, hydrogen and nitrogen. The amino acids are then absorbed into the system where they are re-constituted into amino acid chains that make up cells of the body, like enzymes and hormones. When you consume too much protein, the body has to dispose of the unneeded amino acid chains, and it does this by converting them to carbohydrate or fat. Fat and carbohydrate are comprised of oxygen, hydrogen and carbon; what differentiates protein from fats and carbohydrates is nitrogen.

The conversion of protein into fats and carbohydrate is performed with the assistance of the liver. The carbohydrate is burned for energy or stored as glycogen, and the fat is stored for future use. In order to accomplish this conversion, the nitrogen must be released, which causes the production of ammonia. The ammonia is converted into waste products like urea, uric acid and creatinine, which are disposed of by the kidneys. Excess protein consumption therefore places stress on the liver and kidneys.

Dr. Campbell's research using lab animals at Cornell showed that plant proteins like soy and gluten did not have the same cancer-promoting effects that animal proteins had. However, I have two concerns about excess plant protein consumption. The first is that the body uses complex carbohydrate for energy. Many people are consuming enough calories daily, but are not consuming enough carbohydrate to provide adequate energy for the day's activities because too much protein and fat consumption crowds out carbohydrate consumption. The other concern is that plant proteins contain nitrogen, just as animal protein does, and the body has to clear it, which still results in stress on the liver and kidneys.

The best diet for health maintenance is a near-vegetarian or vegan diet with 75% of calories from complex carbohydrate, 10% of calories as the upper limit from protein and 15% as the upper limit from fat.

Dietary Supplements

As interest in health has increased, Americans' use of dietary supplements has increased too. Most people think that supplements are "natural" and therefore can cause little harm; lots of people think that the worst case scenario with supplements is that they *might* be wasting their money. Few people know that there can be adverse health effects resulting from the use of supplements.

Supplement sellers and some health care practitioners insist that people *need* to take supplements, claiming that people are suffering from deficiencies of certain nutrients like vitamins and minerals. But the reality is that clinical vitamin and other nutrient deficiencies are unusual in Westernized countries. Instead, most people are suffering from diseases of excess; *too much* fat, *too much* protein, *too many* calories. By adopting a plan of dietary excellence as described in this book, the problem of "excess" resolves and an individual can be assured of getting the nutrients needed for optimal human function daily.

Whole Foods are Better

Human bodies require all of the currently known nutrients, as well as those nutrients not yet discovered in food, for proper function. Only a few decades ago, vitamins *themselves* were unknown. New discoveries about nutrients are being made regularly. We now know that there are tens of thousands of constituents in food. None of these substances when separated from the food source can be expected to produce the same result as when they are consumed in nature's perfect packages – food!

Nutrients in food are synergistic; the whole is greater than the sum of its parts. It is illogical to think that isolated nutrients can perform in the same way as whole foods, just as listening to someone playing the clarinet will never be the same as listening to the entire orchestra.

One of my major objections to taking supplements is that the decision to take dietary supplements (for which there is little evidence of benefit and considerable evidence of harm) often postpones or even precludes a decision to adopt a program of dietary excellence (for which there is overwhelming evidence of benefit and no evidence of harm).

Testing for Deficiencies

When medical professionals take blood samples and determine that a person is deficient in vitamins B, C, and E, magnesium, and calcium, these deficiencies are identified because those were the nutrients for which the patient was tested. A person who has low levels of these nutrients is also likely to be deficient in indole-3-carbinole, resveratrol, sulphoraphane, and anthocyanins, as well as thousands of other nutrients, but we don't test for them. The most likely reason for deficiency is poor diet, and the true deficiency is one of whole plant foods, which can only be remedied by converting to a whole-foods, plant-based diet.

There are other issues with testing. These include the fact that human biochemistry changes from day to day, and sometimes even from minute to minute. Tests evaluate nutrient status at a specific moment in time, which may not be indicative of an individual's overall nutrient status.

Testing humans for anything, ranging from nutrient levels to cholesterol, involves interpreting results by comparing individuals with standards set by government agencies or professional organizations, which have often proven to be arbitrary and incorrect.

For example, some doctors still insist that low levels of HDL cholesterol are dangerous; however research shows that total cholesterol and LDL levels are more important than HDL levels. We now know that the body produces less HDL when LDL levels drop, since less of it is needed in order to clear LDL from the bloodstream. At one time, it was thought that blood cholesterol levels of under 150 mg/dl were dangerous; however data gathered as part of the China Project identified healthy rural Chinese with cholesterol levels as low as 80 mg/dl.[70]

The point is that we cannot be certain that optimal nutrient levels have been established; and there is scant evidence to indicate that raising nutrient levels through supplementation is beneficial or improves health outcomes.

The National Academy of Sciences and the Institute of Medicine are responsible for setting daily reference intakes for nutrients. At this time, daily reference intakes have been established for only 25 nutrients, and over the years, changes have been made for several of them based on new research findings.

It is very important to look for true cause and effect relationships when making decisions about taking supplements, or any decision about nutrition, health, and medical care. One key is to understand the difference between *correlation* and *causation*. Correlations are relationships between two factors. For example, some studies show that people who have heart attacks have lower levels of vitamin C. But this does not mean that the *cause* of heart disease is lower levels of vitamin C. We know that all people with lower vitamin C levels do not develop heart disease.

It is quite probable that a lower level of vitamin C is not a risk factor for heart disease by itself but rather a marker for a poor diet, which often *is* a risk factor. The solution, therefore, is not to supplement with vitamin C, but rather to adopt a program of dietary excellence which will not only resolve the vitamin C "deficiency," but also reduce the risk of most common degenerative conditions, including heart disease.

Why are People Still Being Told To Take Supplements?

How did isolated nutrient supplements become so popular? The reason is the way traditional medical practice is structured. Western medicine focuses on treating symptoms with drugs, procedures and surgery. The drugs are very specific and act on the body in very specific ways, like magic bullets. Have a headache? Take an aspirin and it's gone quickly. Have an infection? Take an antibiotic. Getting infections frequently? Take antibiotics frequently. Few doctors take the time to find out *why* a patient has developed a health condition in order to treat the *cause,* which is most likely poor diet and lifestyle. Change the diet and lifestyle in the right ways, and the health conditions usually resolve.

The same philosophy has carried over to the nutrition field. The fascination with individual nutrients is based on medicine's propensity to use specific substances to treat symptoms, rather than diet and lifestyle changes to treat the underlying cause of disease.

When physicians and scientists began observing that people with certain diseases had lower levels of some nutrients in their bloodstream, they assumed a cause and effect relationship. They hypothesized that taking those nutrients in supplement form would raise nutrient levels and therefore lead to health improvement. This approach has led to research focusing on isolated nutrients, trying to duplicate the medical model that has become so familiar. Instead of looking at the totality of the diet, many medical professionals are looking for drug-like nutritional magic bullets to treat disease. The supplements may, in some instances, be less toxic than the drugs, and in some cases, biomarkers are improved. But supplements do not stop the progression of or reverse the disease, and the patient will continue to get sicker over time, even while taking them.

Don't Confuse Feeling Better With Getting Better

Isolated nutrient supplements often "work" in the sense that they may improve symptoms in the short term, but they do not address the underlying causes of illness.

Many people report that they feel better as a result of taking vitamins. But it is important to differentiate between feeling better and getting better. Many people felt better while taking Vioxx for arthritis pain, but some reports estimate that 58,000 people died as a result of taking it.[71] Glucosamine (a dietary supplement derived from the shells of crustaceans), is effective in relieving pain from arthritis in some people. But a diet based on whole plant foods is effective for not only relieving the pain of arthritis, but also for stopping its progression and often even for reversing it. Using diet as the intervention tool causes one to feel better *while* getting better, a much better choice and an important distinction.

This is why research on isolated nutrient supplements, while sometimes producing short-term improvements in symptoms or biomarkers, continually produces disappointing results when evaluated for prevention or long-term health improvement. On the other hand, research on certain dietary intervention protocols, like a low-fat plant-based diet, continues to show that conditions like coronary artery disease and type 2 diabetes can often be stopped or reversed, and patients thrive in the long-term.

Research Continues to Focus on Supplements Instead of Whole Foods and Diet

More research is conducted on the use of isolated nutrients vs. whole foods and dietary patterns. Why? There are several reasons, but one is the way that scientific research is viewed by researchers and the medical community. Most scientists believe that the double-blind placebo-controlled study is the gold standard for research. In these studies, the researchers do not know who is getting the drug or the supplement vs. the placebo. This is thought by most to offer the most potential for objectivity.

But there are limits to using only this research methodology when investigating the effects of diet on health. Obviously, people know what they are eating and so do their observers, making a double-blind placebo- controlled study examining dietary patterns almost impossible to do.

Another important factor that prevents the study of complete dietary protocols like the one I recommend is the bias that many doctors and researchers have about dietary change. The prevailing "wisdom" about dietary excellence is that people will not willingly adopt such a diet, and that even if they do, they will not stick with it.

This is not true. Tens of thousands of people have adopted and maintained a plant-based diet through programs offered by The Wellness Forum, The Physicians Committee for Responsible

Medicine, Dr. Caldwell Esselstyn, Dr. John McDougall, Dr. Alan Goldhamer and many others.

Research has even shown that once people do make these changes, they are quite satisfied with their new diets and generally remain compliant. Although this might sound counterintuitive to some, the reason is that when people make significant changes, their health improves significantly too, which provides a powerful motivator for continuing to be compliant.[72] [73]

The perception of the medical community that people don't want to hear about comprehensive dietary change or are unwilling to make such changes is incorrect. My experience in delivering public lectures and with our growing membership at The Wellness Forum is that there is incredible interest in diet and health; people really are looking for alternative solutions to their health issues.

What About Studies Showing Efficacy of Supplements?

Promoters of vitamins and isolated nutrient supplements point to studies showing that their products are effective. However, the studies are generally for short periods of time and evaluate positive effects on one or two biomarkers. The artificial manipulation of these "surrogate markers" has not generally been shown to improve health, longevity, or quality of life. This is true of both supplements and drugs. Patients often lower their cholesterol, blood sugar levels, or blood pressure with drugs and/or supplements, only to find that they still have progressing heart disease, diabetes and other degenerative conditions. Oncologists often justify the use of certain chemotherapy drugs because the drugs reduce tumors within 30 days, but for many forms of cancer, the patients die only a few months later, making those short-term results irrelevant.

The people who join The Wellness Forum are interested in many years of healthy living, not a temporary improvement in a biomarker followed by declining health or death. It is only by addressing the totality of the diet and lifestyle that long-term health can be achieved.

Disappointing Results

While researchers have noted for years that people who eat more fruits and vegetables have lower risks of diseases like colon cancer and heart disease, studies using antioxidants isolated from fruits and vegetables have produced dismal results.

One of the largest analyses of studies examining the use of antioxidant supplements was conducted by the Cochrane Collaboration.[74] This review included 67 randomized trials with 232,550 participants. Twenty-one trials collectively included 164,439 healthy individuals; the other forty-six trials included 68,111 patients who had various diseases.

The researchers concluded, "We found no evidence to support antioxidant supplements for primary or secondary prevention. Vitamin A, beta-carotene, and vitamin E may increase mortality. Future randomized trials could evaluate the potential effects of vitamin C and selenium for primary and secondary prevention. Such trials should be closely monitored for potential harmful effects. Antioxidant supplements need to be considered medicinal products and should undergo sufficient evaluation before marketing."

Many other studies have reached similar conclusions; that taking isolated antioxidants does not decrease the risk of disease. For example, subjects taking beta carotene, Vitamin C, and alpha-tocopherol did not have lower risks of colon cancer than those taking a placebo.[75]

A study published in *The Journal of the American Medical Association* showed that taking Vitamins C and E did not reduce the risk of heart disease. There was no reduction in the rate of nonfatal myocardial infarction, stroke, cardiovascular death, congestive heart failure, angina or all-cause mortality in the group taking the supplements as compared to those taking placebo. The same study also showed that the supplements did not reduce the risk of cancer.[76]

The *Folate After Coronary Intervention Trial* included 626 patients who had stents implanted in blocked arteries. Half were randomly given folic acid; the other half a placebo. Six months later the arteries of those taking folic acid had narrowed *more* than those taking the placebo.[77]

A study published in the *Journal of the American Medical Association* showed that lowering homocysteine levels by taking supplemental B vitamins did not improve cardiovascular health. After about seven years of follow-up there were no differences in the number of women experiencing cardiovascular events between the group taking B vitamins and the group taking a placebo.[78]

This study and others like it have been conducted in response to evidence that B vitamins lower homocysteine levels (they do); and that higher homocysteine levels are correlated with increased risk of cardiovascular disease (they are). Therefore, researchers assumed, lowering homocysteine levels through supplementation with B vitamins should reduce the risk of cardiovascular disease. The problem is that studies have not proven this hypothesis.

Studies continue to show that the manipulation of biomarkers, either through the use of drugs or supplements, does not improve health outcomes. The reason is clear: taking vitamins does not address the cause of heart attacks and strokes, which is the excessive amount of fat, animal protein and processed junk foods consumed in the Western diet.

There are Risks Associated with Taking Some Supplements!

Some studies have been prematurely ended due to increased incidence of disease or worsening health in the supplement-taking group. This was the case in the SELECT trial (the Selenium and Vitamin E Cancer Prevention Trial), which was stopped by the National Cancer Institute. This study involved 35,534 men age 50 or older taking vitamin E, selenium, a combination of both or a placebo.

A review of the data conducted in September and October 2008 showed that selenium and vitamin E supplements, taken either alone or in combination for five years, did not prevent prostate cancer in the intervention group. The data also showed a small increase in the number of prostate cancer deaths in men taking only vitamin E, and a small increase in the number of men developing diabetes who were taking only selenium. The men were instructed to stop taking their supplements.[79]

What About Vitamin B12?

Although there are good reasons to be cautious about supplements, the one exception may be vitamin B12, particularly for vegans who do not consume any fortified foods.

Vitamin B12 is essential for the health of the nervous system, is needed for the formation of red blood cells, and stimulates growth and appetite in children. It also facilitates the utilization of protein, fat, and carbohydrate; assists in the utilization of iron; and is important for the synthesis of DNA and RNA.

Vitamin B12 is made from bacteria. Humans have historically consumed it in drinking water and other natural sources. One of the great advances of civilization has been cleaning up the water supply so people no longer die from water-borne diseases, and other general improvements in sanitation. But this sterile (and I agree safer) environment results in less B12 being available for human consumption.

Animal foods contain B12 because animals consume bacteria in the plants they eat for food. Gastrointestinal fermentation results in the production of vitamin B12, which is then stored in animal flesh and fat; humans consume it when they eat animal foods.

B12 enters the stomach as part of animal food and is separated from it by digestive enzymes and hydrochloric acid. B12 is also consumed in fortified foods like cereals and plant milks.

Very small amounts of vitamin B12 are needed daily – only 2-4 mcg per day for adults; slightly more for pregnant or lactating women.

The principal food sources of B12 are animal foods such as fish, meat, and eggs. Plant foods do not contain much vitamin B12, but even strict vegans rarely develop B12 deficiencies because most of them consume some vitamin B12 in fortified foods.

There is a general misunderstanding about the B12 content in vegetarian foods like brewer's yeast, fermented soy foods, and sea vegetables. Soy foods contain no measurable amounts of B12. Brewer's yeast generally contains vitamin B12 only if it is fortified with it, and the consumption of fortified and adulterated brewer's yeast is not recommended. Sea vegetables like spirulina actually contain compounds similar to B12 called analogues, making sea vegetables an unreliable source. Some bacteria in the intestine produce vitamin B12, but the amount produced is not enough to prevent deficiency.

Most B12 deficiencies do not develop as a result of inadequate intake, however. Absorption of B12 is dependent on a protein secreted by the stomach called intrinsic factor. This is a binding protein that, when combined with B12, creates a complex that is absorbed in the small intestine. Adequate hydrochloric acid is needed for production of intrinsic factor; decreased hydrochloric acid production results from taking antacids, used frequently by Americans.

Aging, stress, and digestive problems can weaken the body's ability to produce intrinsic factor, and poor intestinal health can result in decreased B12 absorption.
Therefore, B12 deficiency can result even when intake levels are adequate.

The body stores vitamin B12, so deficiencies take many years to develop. The highest concentrations are found in the liver, heart, kidney, pancreas, brain, blood, and bone marrow.

There are no known toxic effects of consuming large doses of B12. But there are serious problems associated with deficiency. These include unusual fatigue, anemia, digestive problems, loss of appetite, anxiety, diarrhea, depression, frequent infections, and nervous system disorders. Numbness and tingling in the hands and feet are often the first to present, since B12 nourishes the myelin sheath that protects the nerves and assists in maintaining electrical conductivity. Other signs of B12 deficiency include soreness and weakness in the arms and legs, decreased sensory perceptions, difficulty in walking and speaking, and neuritis.

Pernicious anemia refers to a condition in which the body does not have enough red blood cells or hemoglobin. It is brought about by persistent impairment in the production of intrinsic factor or inadequate B12 absorption. Fatigue and increasing weakness are common symptoms, and menstrual problems can occur in chronically B12-deficient women.

A B12 deficiency is easily remedied with supplementation; individuals with pernicious anemia may require intramuscular injections. Long-term deficiency conditions can cause permanent damage that is not reparable with supplementation, so it is important to have a blood test performed if you begin to experience any of the symptoms listed above.

The best option is to prevent deficiencies from developing. First, make sure your gastrointestinal tract is working properly. Reflux, gas, bloating, diarrhea, constipation and other forms of discomfort are signs that your GI tract needs help. Taking antacids, laxatives or binding agents relieves symptoms but does not remedy the problem. Consult with a health care practitioner who is experienced at reversing such conditions and adopt a program of dietary excellence.

If you are a strict vegan and consume no fortified foods, take a B12 supplement as an insurance policy.

What About Vitamin D?

Many health professionals are now testing patients for blood levels of vitamin D, and insist that most of their patients are deficient and require supplementation. Their reasoning is that patients with conditions like autoimmune diseases and cancer have been found to have low vitamin D levels, and that supplementation is protective.

I am convinced, and research supports my position, that optimal vitamin D levels have been exaggerated; that "low" vitamin D levels have not been established as a cause for disease; and that oral supplementation is not advisable for most people.

Vitamin D is important - it promotes calcium absorption, assists in calcium deposition in the bones, and helps to regulate blood calcium levels. It is crucial for the maintenance of a healthy nervous system, development of muscle tone, muscle contractions, immune function, the production of insulin, and many other functions.

So far, ten compounds have been identified with Vitamin D characteristics. Vitamin D2, called ergocalciferol, is found in principally in fortified foods and supplements. Vitamin D3, or cholecalciferol, is produced in response to sunlight exposure. A synthetic version of vitamin D is used as a supplement and for fortifying foods like milk. Vitamin D consumed orally requires fat for absorption, but is often added to low-fat milk products or taken alone in supplement form. This may affect absorption and utilization of supplemental D.

The body is designed to produce vitamin D as a result of exposure to sunlight, which means that it should be classified as a hormone rather than a vitamin. Many people do not spend much time outdoors, and some are worried that any sun exposure at all will increase their risk of skin cancer. But sun exposure is necessary for the natural production of vitamin D.

Sun exposure activates a precursor, a form of cholesterol, in the skin and converts it to vitamin D3. Vitamin D made by the skin and not immediately used is stored in the liver, skin, brain, bones, and other tissues. This stored form of vitamin D must be converted to its active form. The process starts in the liver, where it is converted to 25-hydroxy vitamin D, and continues in the kidney where it is converted to 1,25 dihydroxy Vitamin D, or calcitriol.

The conversion of the storage form of vitamin D to its active form is influenced by many factors. The consumption of animal protein causes a significant drop in 1,25 D levels by creating an acidic environment that impairs the action of the kidney enzyme that assists in converting it.

Calcium levels also affect the activity of vitamin D. Higher blood levels of calcium result in a reduction in both the activity of the kidney enzyme needed to convert vitamin D to its active form, and the activity of 1,25D itself. Higher blood calcium levels can result from supplementation, or from the body releasing calcium, a natural buffer, from the bones in order to neutralize the acid load created by eating a diet high in animal protein, fat, processed foods, caffeine, alcohol and other commonly consumed foods. This means that people consuming some version of the Standard American Diet should expect to have lower blood levels of 1,25 D.

Kidney or liver disease can also impair the conversion of stored vitamin D to its active form.

There are differing opinions as to optimal serum levels of vitamin D, which range from 30 to 80 nn/ml. Vitamin D deficiency is generally defined as a level of less than 20 nn/ml, and vitamin D insufficiency as 21 to 29 nn/ml. But a committee appointed by the Institute of Medicine issued a report in 2010 concluding that optimal vitamin D levels are between 20 nn/ml; that most Americans are within that range and able to maintain those levels through sunlight exposure; and that vitamin D supplementation was not advisable.[80] This report analyzed close to 1000 studies examining calcium and vitamin D to determine how much was required and how much was too much. Yet most health care professionals will recommend vitamin D supplementation in response to levels of 30 nn/ml or lower.

Get Out in the Sun!

How much sun exposure is needed in order to produce adequate vitamin D? It is important to get some sun exposure every day possible *without the use of sunscreen*. If you live in a northern climate, start early in the season with exposure for short periods of time; you can remain in the sun until the skin turns pink, as long as it does not burn. If you're planning to be in the sun for longer periods of time, you should wear loose protective clothing and hats.

The amount of time spent in the sun should gradually increase over the summer months; the body stores vitamin D for use during the winter months.

Vitamin D and Disease

Many health care practitioners continue to insist that lower vitamin D levels are related to the development of conditions ranging from depression to cancer. It is true that people with many diseases do seem to have lower blood levels of vitamin D. Are these lower levels the cause of these conditions?

This does not seem to be the case. Animal protein consumption results in an increase in the production of insulin-like growth factor (IGF-1), which can cause abnormal cell proliferation, or cancer. As mentioned earlier, the consumption of animal protein also interferes with the body's ability to convert the storage form of vitamin D to its active form.   It may be that lower vitamin D levels are not the *cause* of cancer, but simply markers for dietary patterns that increase the risk of cancer significantly. In other words, low vitamin D levels may be *correlated* to cancer incidence, but not be the *cause* of cancer.

The aforementioned Institute of Medicine's committee agreed, stating that claims that lower vitamin D levels cause disease "are not supported by the available evidence." The committee found that these claims were based on observations and that there has been no credible research establishing a cause and effect relationship.

Other studies do not support a link either. Researchers at the National Cancer Institute measured the vitamin D levels of 17,000 people. Ten years after the study began, 536 people had died of cancer. There was no correlation between vitamin D levels and the risk of dying of cancer.[81]

Another study, the RECORD trial, involved 5,292 patients who were enrolled through 21 health centers in England and Scotland. The participants were randomized to receive 800 IU of vitamin D, 1000 mg calcium, both, or placebo; and then followed for 24-62 months. The study was conducted to assess the relationship between vitamin D deficiency and insulin production, and to determine if insulin production could be increased with vitamin D supplementation.

The researchers found no evidence that supplementation with vitamin D, either alone or with calcium, prevented the development of diabetes or reduced medication levels for diabetics.[82]

Michael Hollick, M.D., Ph.D., is a highly respected researcher and an expert on vitamin D. He is a professor of medicine and physiology, and formerly of dermatology, at Boston University School of Medicine, and (until 2000) chief of endocrinology, metabolism and nutrition.

According to Dr. Hollick, oral supplementation is an inefficient way to increase vitamin D levels. Dr. Hollick instead recommends sun exposure. He says that just 10-15 minutes in the sun is the equivalent of taking between 15,000 and 20,000 IU's of vitamin D, but without the potential for toxicity that is becoming more common as people take larger doses of it orally.[83]

There is a difference between vitamin D synthesized from the sun and vitamin D taken orally, since there are additional photoproducts made in response to sun exposure that are not in the supplement form of vitamin D. That means that it is important to enable the body to *make* vitamin D rather than to *supplement* with it.

As is the case with so many isolated nutrients, there are risks associated with taking vitamin D supplements. For example, men may increase their risk of prostate cancer by taking vitamin D supplements.[84]

And vitamin D supplements given to women were shown to increase their "bad" LDL cholesterol by 4.1% and reduce their HDL/LDL ratio by 10.5%.[85] Supplements and fortified milk have caused toxic effects in some people.[86]

And the Institute of Medicine report concurred, stating that supplementation leading to higher levels of vitamin D can increase the risk of fracture, disease, and all-cause mortality. The committee also wrote that while studies were not conclusive, that vitamin D supplements were not a good idea in the absence of proven benefit. The committee found evidence "challenging the concept that 'more is better.'

In conclusion, the current body of research does not support the idea that most people are deficient in vitamin D; that lower vitamin D levels are the cause of disease; or that supplementation is safe or effective.

Sunlight exposure and dietary excellence™ are the best ways to insure adequate blood levels of vitamin D.

The Proper Use of Supplements

Is there ever a proper use for isolated nutrient supplements? Yes – in a clinical setting. For example, high-quality, high-potency probiotics are necessary for restoring gut flora following an antibiotic regimen, and can be helpful in treating many gastrointestinal disorders.

There have been some excellent results documented for using high-dose nutrient supplements or nutrients delivered via IV as adjuvant, or complementary treatments for conditions like cancer. And there are constructive ways in which supplements can be used to promote more rapid recovery while patients improve their diet and lifestyle.

The important thing to remember is that isolated nutrients often have pharmacological effects, and therefore should be respected like medicines. They can cause side effects, making self-medication with them a bad idea. Supplements that are effective for treating mild to moderate depression, for example, are contraindicated for people who are taking many commonly-prescribed pharmaceutical antidepressants. And some supplements are not safe for pregnant women. When supplements are called for, they should be taken under the direction of a knowledgeable professional who is properly trained, and almost always for short periods of time. In addition, a program of dietary excellence™ and optimal habits should be adopted to resolve the underlying condition.

It is true that food itself is medicine. The science simply does not support the use of isolated nutrient supplements as a substitute for food for achieving or maintaining optimal health. The incredible stories of healing that you will read about later in this book were not achieved with dietary supplements; they were the result of dietary excellence™.

Confusing Information

During the last several decades a very important shift has taken place in the world. We now have access to more information about almost everything, including health, than we have ever had in the past. People are more interested in disease prevention, nutrition, and healthcare than ever before, and more of them are doing their own research because they want to be more in charge of their health. Many patients are unwilling to allow health care professionals to make decisions for them and to just do what they are told. For the most part, this is a good thing.

Newspapers, magazines, television, and the internet provide enormous amounts of information on diet, health and medicine every day. The problem is that although some of the information is excellent, much of it is questionable, and a lot of it is incorrect. The dilemma for the average person is sorting it all out; figuring out which sources are reliable and which information is accurate. This is not easy, even for well-educated people.

An entire industry has developed around the dissemination of health information through books, tapes, television shows, and the media. One of my pet peeves is the growing number of health care professionals who make their entire living as health experts/media personalities. Many of these individuals have never conducted scientific research; some do not currently treat patients and many never have. Although they understand health issues because of their education, their lack of research or clinical experience often results in the dispensing of incorrect advice.

Other so-called "health experts" have no training at all. Some are celebrities, and many are being paid to endorse products or programs. They have no credentials that qualify them to evaluate information or to make recommendations about nutrition and health. But they generate a lot of attention and it is not uncommon for millions of people to buy their books and products, and to follow their advice. Some of their appeal is based on their anti-medical establishment views. While we might all agree that traditional approaches to health are ineffective, it does not follow that all non-traditional approaches to health are well-researched and scientifically proven.

To add to the confusion generated by the media, professional experts and celebrities, there are problems with both the structure of studies that look at diet and health and how the results of these studies are reported to the public.

Structuring Diet Studies is Difficult

One of the biggest issues that plagues scientific research on diet and health is that so much research involves studies that look at the effects of a single nutrient or food rather than examining the effects of dietary pattern on health. This is a very important limitation in view of the fact that both population studies and the results produced by doctors who are stopping the progression of or reversing disease have all achieved success with *total dietary change*, not with single nutrients or foods.

But designing studies that look at diet and lifestyle is a difficult task. People, even those who live in the same area, are members of the same ethnic group, or share certain characteristics, such as socioeconomic status, are very different. Their diets may be similar but have minor, yet important variables. This can make it difficult both to structure a study and to draw conclusions from the data gathered.

Another issue is the time period for which study participants are followed, and the outcomes being tracked. Sometimes research shows a short-term positive effect for a particular food or nutrient, but it becomes quite meaningless in the long term. This phenomenon also affects drug research. Many cancer drugs that reduce the size of tumors within a few weeks do not extend life; the short term result of tumor reduction means nothing in terms of long-term health and survival. And so it is with foods and nutrients. A diet that "works" in the short-term for weight loss, such as the Atkins diet, causes bone loss, heart disease and rebound weight gain in the long term, making the short-term results, even if they are positive, meaningless.

The financial resources required for tracking people and their diets over long periods of time are significant and often unavailable; the larger the number of participants and the more variables included, the more expensive the study will be.

Even when adequate funding is available, tracking the effects of diet on health is very difficult. Subjects are given a dietary protocol, sometimes with training and sometimes without, and then have to try to stick with it on their own. In many studies, subjects self-report. Researchers acknowledge serious limitations in self-reporting; without intending to do so, subjects will often misrepresent their eating patterns. People have difficulty remembering what they ate; let's face it – most of us would have trouble recalling what we ate last week with any degree of accuracy. They often report consuming more healthy foods like fruit and vegetables, and are reluctant to report desserts, snacks, and foods that make their dietary patterns look bad.[87] This, to a certain extent, is human nature. Even slight variations can significantly change research conclusions.

There are lots of studies that have looked at the relationship between diet and health in which none of the participants or groups were eating a health-promoting diet, or in which the dietary changes that were made were so small as to be insignificant. The poor design of these studies can significantly affect the results and lead to gross misconceptions.

People can also be misled by reading the results of a single study. With all well-researched topics, not all studies show the same findings. There are studies, for example, that show that smoking does not increase the risk of developing lung cancer. But *most* studies do. This is why it is important not to place a lot of emphasis on only one study – its conclusions may not represent what most of the evidence shows on a particular topic.

In order to get to the truth about diet and health, many studies should be reviewed, those with poor design should be set aside, and conclusions should be drawn based on the preponderance of the evidence. A meta-analysis is designed to do just that - it uses data from several studies to combine the data into one set. If they are well-constructed, these studies are generally more reliable than single studies. Problems can develop even with meta-analyses, however, if the selection criteria for the studies are incorrect or skewed by industry influence or other pressures.

This does not mean that research cannot help us to determine the best diet for humans, or that we don't have enough research to make solid recommendations. But it may help you to understand why you see so much conflicting information in the media daily and why more scientists are not advocating a plant-based diet like the one I am recommending.

In order to illustrate these points, I've included reviews of a few studies that, while they have attracted a lot of attention, are quite misleading.

Vegetarians do not Live Longer than Meat-Eaters

In March 2009, the *American Journal of Clinical Nutrition*[88] reported the results of a study showing that vegetarians do not live longer than meat eaters. How could this be? If a plant-based diet reduces the risk of degenerative disease, and these diseases are the cause of most deaths, shouldn't the plant eaters be living longer?

This study summarized the results of five prospective studies that enrolled vegetarians and non-vegetarians with similar lifestyles. The researchers sought to find out whether or not vegetarians had lower mortality rates from ischemic heart disease, and colorectal, breast, and prostate cancers.

In one study, vegetarians were people who replied "yes" to the question "Are you a vegetarian?" In the four other studies vegetarians were defined as people who said that they did not eat any meat or fish; all others were labeled "non-vegetarians."

There were two problems with the selection of the subjects. The first is the definition of "vegetarian." People who define themselves as vegetarians because they eat no meat or fish are often still consuming large amounts of dairy products and eggs. Continuing to consume moderate to large amounts of animal protein from sources other than meat and fish will not result in health improvement.

98

As for the vegan subjects, while the elimination of meat, dairy, and fish from the diet can be an important first step toward health improvement, much more dietary modification is needed in order to achieve optimal health. There are lots of near-vegetarians and vegans who consume diets high in fats and oils and highly processed and refined foods. They often remain overweight and continue to experience health issues because their diets are far from ideal.

Based on these selection criteria, the conclusion that these loosely defined "vegetarians" do not live longer than meat eaters is not surprising. People who do not practice dietary excellence, regardless of whether they do or do not eat animal foods, do not experience optimal health or have reduced risks of developing degenerative diseases.

In defense of the researchers who conducted this study, it is difficult to recruit a large cohort of people who practice dietary excellence in order to compare outcomes in a meaningful way. But it is important to keep this in mind when reviewing results of studies evaluating diet and health.

Vegetarian Diet Weakens Bones

Yahoo News Canada featured an article in mid-2009 titled "Vegetarian Diet Weakens Bones." The article began with this statement, "People who live on vegetarian diets have slightly weaker bones than their meat-eating counterparts..."

A Malaysian dairy producer and wholesaler, AMBer Alliance Inc, funded this study. This was not mentioned in any of the news articles I was able to find when I conducted an internet search.

The study was a meta-analysis of nine studies, which were selected from a total of 922 studies. [89] As I mentioned earlier, meta-analyses can sometimes be helpful in drawing conclusions about research, but selection criteria designed to choose only nine studies from such a large body of research is concerning; it is unlikely that this meta-analysis represents the preponderance of the evidence.

More important, however, was that the results of the study were virtually meaningless. The study concluded that the bones of vegetarians were 5% less dense the bones of those who consumed animal foods; for vegans the difference was 6%. Lead researcher Tuan Nguyen stated himself that although the study showed that vegetarian and vegan diets are associated with lower bone mineral density, *"the magnitude of the association is clinically insignificant."* (emphasis mine)

The study showed no correlation between dietary calcium intake and bone mineral density. But even the inclusion of this measurement is meaningless; bone mineral density is a poor determinant of the risk of fracture.[90]

In other words, a study funded by a dairy producer showed a clinically insignificant difference between the bone mineral density (a meaningless biomarker) of vegetarians, vegans and people who consume animal foods.

So why did this study get any attention at all? I cannot confirm this, but the dairy producer that funded the study may have generated the publicity about it. This is a common practice for food companies and agricultural organizations anxious to show that their products are beneficial for health.

Reporters are often not very knowledgeable about health and how to read studies; they will simply report what they are told. Great for industry, not so great for the average consumer who believes information presented in the media.

Confusing Research Findings
About Diet and Cancer

The Journal of the National Cancer Institute published an article online[91] in which researchers reported that eating more servings of fruits and vegetables daily did not significantly reduce the risk of cancer.

Researchers obtained data on 478,478 men and women in ten European countries and then followed them for an average of 8.7 years. They assessed the association between cancer risk and fruit and vegetable consumption. The researchers concluded that "high intake of vegetables, and fruits and vegetables combined, was associated with a small reduction in overall cancer risk."

I'm not surprised at these results, and I actually agree with the findings of the researchers. The problem is not that the conclusions are incorrect; the problem is study design, and the interpretation and reporting of the results, which are very misleading.

The term "high intake" as applied to the fruit and vegetable consumption of the study participants might lead one to believe that the participants were eating a plant-based diet. But this was not the case.

Scientific American included this comment in its online article covering the study: "The researchers concluded that if the results of the analysis can be broadly applied, upping daily fruit and vegetable consumption by about 150 grams (equivalent to about one cup of cherry tomatoes or 1.5 medium bananas), from most dietary levels, could prevent about 2.5% of cancers in most populations." This is true; an extra serving of vegetables or fruit daily is not enough to improve anyone's health outcomes substantially.

This study's structure and conclusions are examples of the problems I described earlier. Scientists tend to structure studies that evaluate the effects of individual nutrients or foods, or small variations in less-than-optimal diets on health, instead of looking at the totality of the diet, or insisting on comparing outcomes from significantly different diets. This is a very important limiting factor.

Those of us who are recommending a well-structured plant-based diet as a means for preventing, stopping the progression of, and even reversing disease, are achieving spectacular results by teaching people to make *sweeping changes* in their diets, not by adding or restricting one food, or by making small changes in their eating patterns. These changes include the elimination of dairy products; reducing or eliminating the consumption of all other animal foods (the upper limit being 10% of calories);

reducing fat and eliminating oils; and eating a diet comprised of high-fiber, nutrient-dense, whole plant foods. Studies have shown that such a diet is not only protective, but can actually stop the progression of and even reverse disease.[92] [93] [94]

In this case, the researchers were attempting to isolate the protective effects of what turned out to be very small differences in the amounts of fruits and vegetables consumed on cancer incidence. Although they did factor in consumption of alcohol and smoking, they did not take into consideration other very important dietary factors such as animal protein, which has been proven to be a powerful cancer promoter;[95] dietary fat, including monounsaturated and polyunsaturated fat, which is also a significant factor in cancer risk;[96] and the consumption of dairy products, which has been linked to several forms of cancer, particularly prostate cancer.[97] But these factors were not considered.

The dietary habits in this study were self-reported, and as I mentioned before, researchers acknowledge limitations in self-reported information, as stated earlier.[98]

The unfortunate result of studies of this type is that they confuse people, perpetuating the idea that diseases like cancer are largely unpreventable and that diet does not really matter. This turns people into helpless victims rather than empowering them to take control of their health.

A well-structured plant-based diet *is* effective in reducing the risk of common degenerative diseases, and has been proven to be a powerful tool in helping sick people to regain their health. Much research has already been conducted and published proving this relationship, and medical journals and the media need to report *this* information to the general public.

Lack of Training

A logical place to get information on diet and health should be the doctors' office. Patients often ask their doctors about diet; and doctors know patients are interested in information about nutrition. Some are anxious to give advice because they know that diet does make a difference.

Although it's fair to assume that most people enter the health care field because they want to help people and their intentions are admirable, good intentions cannot overcome poor training, or, in the case of nutrition, a complete lack of training. Most medical schools offer little to no training in nutrition science to doctors. It's no wonder doctors give out inaccurate nutrition advice, cannot evaluate nutrition research, or completely discount the powerful effects of diet on health outcomes!

In the case of dietitians, the problem is their accrediting body, the American Dietetic Association. This organization, which has suffers from serious conflict of interest issues due to its dependence on sponsorships from agricultural groups and food companies, approves the educational curriculum for dietitians and designs and administers testing to certify their competence. While there are many excellent dietitians in practice today, the vast majority are victims of their training, which is focused on the USDA's dietary recommendations, food service operations, and the philosophy that there is a place for all foods in the daily diet (a philosophy that is good for sponsors, but not for public health).

The Wellness Forum Institute for Health Studies is working to change this situation by offering a certificate program for health care practitioners that teaches them how to use diet and lifestyle as a primary intervention tool. The course is taught by the best experts in this area, including Dr. Campbell, Dr. McDougall, Dr. Esselstyn, Dr. Goldhamer, Dr. Moss and others. We are optimistic that this program will help to significantly increase the number of diet-centered providers quickly, since it is unlikely that educational programs for health care professionals will change soon.

We also offer an alternative to traditional dietetics, the Nutrition Educator Program, which includes a strong scientific foundation, and a focus on plant-based nutrition, with no industry influence.

Science vs. Advertising

One of the basic tenants of a democracy is the right to free speech, and this includes the right of companies to advertise their products. Legally, advertisers are bound to make truthful statements when promoting their products, but it is possible to make a statement that may be technically true, but at the same time be incredibly misleading. Food companies are particularly skilled in using claims about individual ingredients in order to make their foods appear to be healthier than they really are. Here are a few examples.

Kashi is marketing a "healthier cracker" fortified with plant sterols that is promoted as the "first nationally distributed cracker to provide more for your heart". Eating Cheerios is advertised on television and in print ads as a way to lower your cholesterol (the fine print states that cholesterol is lowered by 4% in six weeks, an insignificant reduction, but the average person does not read the fine print or understand this issue well). One-hundred-calorie packs of foods like Doritos and offerings such as Oreos Thin Crisps are marketed as a way to help with portion control and calorie reduction.

Pepsi-Co uses a designation called "Smart Spot" that signifies that products have met certain nutritional standards. The problem is that the "standards" are established by Pepsi, which results in this logo appearing on products like Diet Pepsi, Diet Mountain Dew, Baked Cheetos, Doritos, and Lay's Potato Chips.

Kraft has a "Sensible Solution" line of products that contain nutrients such as fiber or calcium, or have lower amounts of fat or sodium than the regular versions of those products. With a product line that includes Kool-Aid and Velveeta Cheese, this designation is virtually meaningless.

Taken at face value these ads promise Americans that they should be able to prevent heart disease by eating crackers and cereal, lose weight while eating Doritos and Oreos, and improve their nutritional status by consuming Diet Mountain Dew and Cheetos. Unfortunately, many members of the public believe these claims and many buy these products expecting to improve their health.

Alliances with national health organizations provide great opportunities for food companies to promote their products too. The average consumer is not aware of the close relationship between these trusted health authorities and food companies, agricultural organizations, and drug companies, but these relationships influence the information they dispense.

The American Diabetes Association is a good example. Although this organization is staffed with many well-meaning people who want to help diabetics, it is almost impossible to give the right advice to the group's diabetic constituents without upsetting its sponsors.

As I mentioned earlier, for several months in 2003, the "Health Tip of the Day" on the ADA's website was sponsored by Eskimo Pie. On April 21, 2005, the American Diabetes Association announced a 3-year multi-million dollar alliance with Cadbury-Schweppes, the third largest soft drink manufacturer in the world, and the maker of the Crème eggs everyone loves to eat at Easter time. We can all agree that diabetics do not need to consume more soft drinks, Eskimo Pies, or Crème Eggs, so how can these relationships possibly benefit diabetic patients?

Perhaps the most egregious examples of advertising disguised through partnership is The American Academy of Family Physicians' Consumer Alliance program. The Coca-Cola Company signed on as the organization's first partner.

The agreement specifies that Coke provide grant money to the AAFP, and in return the AAFP will develop consumer education content on beverages and sweeteners for its website, FamilyDoctor.org. This is terrific – people who want more information about the role of soft drinks and sugar in the diet can now visit the AAFP's website and get information sponsored by Coke.

No wonder Americans are confused!

Industry Funding

The average consumer reading about research results in *USA Today* or *Prevention Magazine* does not know which studies are funded by industry, or about the affiliations of the researchers conducting these studies. One glaring example of the influence funding sources can have on research outcomes is the dairy industry and the millions of dollars it has spent on research showing that consuming dairy products promotes weight loss. Producers and manufacturers of dairy products have aggressively advertised these "research findings" in order to sell their products.

The industry based its campaign on two small studies that were conducted by Michael Zemel, Ph.D., at the University of Tennessee. Dr. Zemel's relationships with dairy associations and private industry are quite interesting. Since 1998, Zemel has received $1.7 million in research grants from the National Dairy Council and $275,000 from General Mills. He has patented a weight-loss program that is now licensed to the International Dairy Foods Association. Advertisers participate in Zemel's "calcium key program" by paying fees that exceed $50,000 a year each.[99] [100]

But according to Amy Lanou, Ph.D., and Neal Barnard, MD, the results of other clinical trials do not support the use of calcium or dairy products for weight or fat loss.[101]

A recent study of 12,829 children showed that the more milk they drank, the more weight they gained. Those consuming more than three servings of dairy products per day were 35% more likely to develop a weight problem than those who consumed only one or two.[102]

The Physicians Committee for Responsible Medicine (PCRM) filed two major lawsuits in 2005 against three dairy industry trade groups—the International Dairy Foods Association, the National Dairy Council, and Dairy Management, Inc., along with Kraft Foods, General Mills, and Dannon. PCRM claimed that these groups were misleading consumers with deceptive advertising about the effect of dairy products on weight loss. McNeill Nutritionals, LLC, the maker of Lactaid; and LifeWay Foods, the manufacturer of a yogurt-like beverage called kefir; were also named as defendants.

In 2007, the Federal Trade Commission ruled that research did not support the claim that dairy helped with weight loss. Lydia Parnes, director of the agency's Bureau of Consumer Protection, reported that Agriculture Department representatives and milk

producers and processors had agreed to change the advertisements and related marketing materials "until further research provides stronger, more conclusive evidence of an association between dairy consumption and weight loss."
In spite of the FTC ruling, articles continue to appear in popular magazines claiming that consuming dairy products will help dieters lose weight.

Disguised Industry Spokespersons

Another ploy used by the food and beverage industry is to set up and/or fund organizations that give the appearance of being independent research groups, but really are just mouthpieces for their industry backers. A good example is the American Council on Science and Health.

The name sounds impressive, and the president, Elizabeth Whelan, has degrees from The Yale School of Medicine and The Harvard School of Public Health. An average consumer might think that Dr. Whelan and her organization would be a good source of information about nutrition and health. And, indeed, Dr. Whelan and the ACSH are regularly consulted by the press and even Congressional committees for expert opinions about nutrition.

The information provided by this group, however, is questionable. In a 2005 article, Dr. Whelan stated that General Mills' ad campaign to get kids to eat their cereals should be praised for its pro-health message. She criticizes individuals who don't think kids should eat sugary cereals, saying "...a parade of churlish nutritionists stepped up to the microphone and complained that General Mills was acting irresponsibly by urging kids to eat cereal that contains sugar...Not only did these critics specifically target the cereals' sugar as a health villain, they went on to suggest that products like Cocoa Puffs contribute to our nation's obesity problem. A number of these naysayers actually went on to say that presweetened cereals were nutritionally worthless..."[103]

Dr. Whelan gushed over the nutritional benefits of Cocoa Puffs for children with this statement: "...the nutrition facts are nonetheless impressive. A one-cup serving offers 25% of your requirements for folic acid, zinc, iron, niacin, vitamin B-12, riboflavin and for other nutrients, you get even more. And you get all this nutrition for only ...160 calories."[104] She admits that 50 of these calories are derived from sugar, but sees nothing wrong with this.

Whelan continued, "Given the fact that most cereals – presweetened or not – are highly nutritious products, why are individuals who boast nutrition training condemning them?"[105] Then she answered her own question by stating, "Food and nutrition issues are poorly understood. In discussions of food – especially as it relates to kids – rational assessments and critical thinking are often abandoned, replaced by closely held but unscientific views. The popular wisdom dictates that sugar is 'bad' although there is no evidence that, when used in moderation like other ingredients, it threatens health or makes kids fat. Sugar simply makes nutritious foods like cereal taste better to kids."

These statements indicate that there is more here than meets the eye. Who *is* the American Council on Science and Health and why would its president make these ridiculous statements?

ACSH was founded by Elizabeth Whelan and Dr. Frederick Stare in 1978. According to Whelan, the organization was organized in response to a request from Pfizer to create a piece addressing the "Delaney Clause" in the 1958 Food Additive Amendment. This clause restricted the use of cancer-causing chemicals in food. Whelan wrote *Panic in the Pantry*, a "book on the history of food scares" that reassured Americans that they did not need to worry about cancer-causing chemicals in food.

Eventually, the organization started seeking financial commitments from other companies. This is when its recommendations became even more blatantly pro-industry. Whelan wrote in a 1981 letter to Senator Henry Waxman that her group opposed government labeling restrictions on additives such as saccharin and nitrites "because there is no adequate data to support the hypotheses that these substances pose a risk to human health." She stated in another interview, "There is room in life for potato chips and twinkies and all these other maligned foods if you don't eat huge amounts of them."

Seventy-six percent of the group's funding comes from corporations and corporate donors according to the National Environmental Trust.[106]

Who are these corporate donors to ACSH? The American Meat Institute, Anheuser Busch Foundation, Burger King, Campbell Soup, Carnation, Coca-Cola, Frito Lay, Hershey Foods, Kellogg Company, Kraft Foundation, M&M Mars, Merck, Oscar Mayer Foods, Pillsbury, and Stouffer are just a few.

As you can see, it is important to know which organizations are providing funding for research, the industry ties of researchers, and the financial backers of those disseminating information to the public in order to determine the validity of the information you are given.

Misrepresentation by the Media

The "Coffee study" is a great example of how writers who are not well-educated about diet and health, or are even just seeking headlines, can mislead people.

A few years ago, newspapers and magazines nationwide featured articles stating that coffee was a good source of antioxidants, implying that coffee might be beneficial for health. Caffeine junkies throughout the US were excited – finally some justification for their daily caffeine fix!

The statements were not entirely true, however. The articles were based on information presented to the American Chemical Society.[107] This information involved the analysis of the antioxidant content of 100 foods and beverages in the American diet and the USDA's estimated per capita consumption of them. At no time did the presenter state that coffee was a health food, or even recommend its consumption. The premise of the presentation was that coffee contains antioxidants, and due to the poor construction of the Standard American Diet, the principal source of antioxidants in the diet for many people has become coffee. Forty-nine percent of Americans are coffee drinkers, who average 3-4 cups a day. This is not so much an advertisement for the health benefits of coffee as it is a report on how terrible the average American's diet really is.

Coffee actually was further down the list in terms of antioxidant content than many other foods. Again, the report was not that coffee was healthy, but that people consume a lot of it.

Lead researcher for the "coffee study," Joe Vinson of the University of Scranton, Pennsylvania, stated, "Unfortunately, consumers are still not eating enough fruits and vegetables, which are better for you from an overall nutritional point of view due to their higher content of vitamins, minerals, and fiber."

He also added that since other studies have implicated coffee as leading to high blood pressure, increased heart rate, stomach pain, and other health problems, more human studies are needed to clarify the impact of coffee on health.

Pressure to Conform

As you can see, the odds of getting accurate information about diet and health from the media or health care professionals are not good. This is further compounded by the fact that the pursuit of scientific truth has ruined or compromised the careers of many. Scientists often find it difficult to pursue research that can lead to the "wrong" conclusions in the eyes of certain groups, and practitioners are often ostracized and sometimes even disciplined if they treat patients with what are considered non-traditional methods.

This situation is not new; people with new ideas about everything ranging from astronomy to the origin of man have been punished for their different views for centuries.

You might think at this point that we all should throw up our hands in despair because the situation is hopeless. But it is not. As I stated in the beginning of this chapter, information is increasingly available to the public, including the information in this book. I am quite optimistic that information about better health through diet and lifestyle change will eventually become available to most Americans. In fact, I am counting on you to help me to spread this message.

Developing Your Health Care Philosophy
and
Choosing Health Care Practitioners

Developing a Personal Health Care Philosophy

Taking the time to develop a personal health care philosophy is a good investment – it allows you to make future choices about medical care within a framework of priorities pre-determined by you.

Following are some items that you might include in your personal health care philosophy:

- I will practice dietary excellence and optimal habits as a means for reducing my risk of degenerative conditions as much as possible.
- When possible, I will hire practitioners who practice dietary excellence and optimal habits, since these people are in the best position to advise me about health issues.
- I will interview health care practitioners prior to retaining them to determine whether or not they share my health care philosophy and are respectful of my views.
- I will limit the number of diagnostic tests I undergo to those that have been proven to be useful, and that are necessary for me.
- Prior to taking any drug or agreeing to any procedure, I will research both the side effects and efficacy rates, and any alternatives to these drugs and procedures.
- I will take the lowest dose of any drug I need to take for the shortest period of time possible.
- I will discontinue my relationship with any health care provider who is not respectful of my philosophy and choices.
- I will not sign any consent form without thoroughly reading and editing it to make sure my intentions are clear.

Choosing your Doctor

The best choice is a doctor who is trained in and committed to practicing Diet-Centered Health Care. A list of doctors and other health care providers who have been trained in this particular type of practice can be accessed at www.wellnessforum.com. The practitioners on this list meet one of two criteria; either they

113

have been successfully using diet as a primary intervention tool for many years, like Dr. McDougall or Dr. Esselstyn, or they have taken The Diet and Lifestyle Intervention Course through The Wellness Forum Institute for Health Studies.

What is Diet-Centered Health Care?

Diet-centered health care is defined as addressing the *cause* of the condition, which is almost always related at least in part, to diet and lifestyle habits, and addressing the cause by *changing* those habits. Practitioners using this approach have become specialists in stopping the progression of or reversing diseases, rather than just treating symptoms with drugs or supplements while the conditions progress and the patients get sicker.

Another key defining characteristic is the amount of time these practitioners spend with their patients in order to insure that they thoroughly understand the cause of their illnesses and how the changes they are being instructed to make will help. For example, membership in The Wellness Forum begins with a 10-hour course during which you learn the science and the skills needed to improve your health. Dr. Caldwell Esselstyn and his wife, Ann, spend several hours with each new patient, and stay in touch regularly to help keep patients on track. Dr. John McDougall offers a 10-day residential program to help his patients adopt a new diet and lifestyle. Rather than just being told what to do, these professionals want patients to understand *why* they are doing it.

Many people in the health care field erroneously assume that patients are not interested in this type of information, but this is not true. Most people find it empowering to learn how their conditions have developed, the influences of diet and lifestyle on their diseases, and what they can do to get better.
An exciting aspect of this type of care is that the patient becomes very involved in his or her own care, and the practitioners and their patients become partners.

Another important point is that these professionals lead by example, which is unfortunately unusual. Although common sense tells us that a practitioner who looks healthy and engages in healthier behaviors is more credible, research actually shows that patients think that doctors who practice healthy habits are more believable and motivating to them.[108]

Professionals certified as diet-centered practitioners acknowledge the importance of other aspects of health, such as exercise, sleep and dealing with stress. However, they all agree with Dr. Esselstyn, who says, "Diet trumps all." The positive effects of meditation and other practices are not to be completely discounted, but they will all tell patients that no one ever meditated their way out of heart disease, and that the influences of stress and other factors on disease development have been grossly over-estimated.

One of Dr. Esselstyn's favorite examples is the rapid drop in deaths from heart disease in Norway during the German occupation in World War II. It's difficult to imagine any situation more stressful than living in a country occupied by Nazi's, yet studies show that deaths from heart disease plummeted during this time and then rapidly increased after the end of the war.[109] How could this be? The explanation is quite interesting. When the Germans occupied a country, they set aside what was considered the best food for the German soldiers – animal foods like steak and chicken. As a result, during the war the Norwegians were forced to live on potatoes and vegetables, their health improved, and the rate of heart disease dropped. As soon as the Germans left, they were able to return to their former diet, and deaths from heart disease began increasing just as rapidly as they had dropped.

Attempts to prevent, stop the progression of, or reverse disease almost always fail until an optimal diet is adopted. Diet-centered practitioners focus on helping patients to make those changes first. They lead by example by not only eating well, but by engaging in regular exercise; leading balanced lives that include family, travel and hobbies; and they encourage their patients to do the same. But they are clear; health improvement is only available to those who practice dietary excellence.™

Choosing a Doctor Not on our List

Although the list of practitioners who are grounded in diet-centered health care is growing and I visualize a day when tens of thousands of providers practice this way, you may be faced with having to find a physician in your area who is not part of our group or trained by us.

Asking friends is a good place to start. Your goal is to find a doctor who will at least listen to you and be respectful of your choices.

Once you have identified a potential doctor, the next step is to schedule a visit. You may choose to make the first visit an interview, rather than an examination. Here are some sample questions you might ask your prospective doctor:

- How much time do you generally spend with your patients?
- How long does it take to get an appointment with you if I have a problem?
- Will you correspond with me via email to answer health care questions?
- What types of diagnostic tests do you recommend to your patients?
- How will you respond if I tell you that I choose not to have a particular test performed?
- I generally do not like to take pharmaceutical drugs, and in the event that I am diagnosed with a condition that does not involve an emergency, might be inclined to seek advice about other options for treatment, such dietary intervention or therapeutic fasting. Are you comfortable with this and can I expect that you will respect my decisions?
- Do you allow pharmaceutical reps to buy lunches, dinners, and to provide other entertainment for you and your staff? Do you teach continuing education programs for pharmaceutical companies? Do you conduct drug trials or other research for drug companies? An affirmative answer would not necessarily eliminate the doctor, but this disclosure would be important as you consider his/her recommendations.

If you have already been diagnosed with a condition and are taking drugs for it, you should ask this question:
"I am now in the process of significantly improving my diet and lifestyle as a means for improving my health. I would like to

discontinue the use of medications as soon as possible, or at the very least, reduce the dosages as much as possible. Will you cooperate with me in doing this?"

You also should ask your prospective doctor about his or her ideas about diet and lifestyle, and how those ideas and philosophy developed. It is often helpful to know which people, books, groups, or organizations are influencing your doctor's thoughts and recommendations.

Based on your decisions to take control of your own health, you're not looking for someone to tell you what to do. You also do not need to find a doctor who agrees with all of your dietary choices or medical decisions. You're looking for someone who will perform diagnostic tests when they are warranted; provide objective information; listen and discuss issues with you; and support your decisions regarding how you choose to take care of yourself.

Annual Physical Exams

Dr. John McDougall frequently cites his own experience to demonstrate how useless these exams can be. In spite of annual physical examinations, after which he was told he was fine, he suffered a stroke at the age of 18, had high cholesterol (335) by age 22, was 50 pounds overweight by the age of 24, and underwent abdominal surgery at the age of 25.

The Canadian Task Force on Periodic Health Examination, the American College of Physicians, the American Medical Association, the US Preventive Services Task Force, and the US Public Health Service have all agreed that routine physical exams for healthy adults are a waste of time and money. Yet, a survey of physicians that appeared in the *Archives of Internal Medicine* in 2005 reported that almost 2/3 of doctors still recommend annual physicals to their patients, and that 2/3 of patients consider the annual physical a medical necessity.[110]

This unwarranted focus on exams is one contributor to our bloated medical system and ever-increasing health insurance costs. Medical care should be reserved for people who require it because they are sick. But people, with ample encouragement from the medical profession, insist on expensive regular physical exams, which as you will learn later in this book, are often followed by useless diagnostic tests and treatments that do not work. The majority of the cost is paid by insurance companies, which makes consumers less conscious of the medical necessity of such visits, tests and treatments.

Doctors and traditional professionals often counter that regular doctor visits and testing lead to early detection, therefore making conditions more treatable, but the reality is that by the time the most deadly conditions are detectable, they are usually quite advanced. The usual treatments do little more than suppress the symptoms rather than addressing the cause of the health condition.

The better alternative would be to meet with a diet-centered health care practitioner to review your diet and lifestyle patterns. Make positive changes in your diet, your weight and body composition, exercise program, your stress levels and the general way in which you are leading your life. This proactive approach gives you the best chance of not getting sick.

Diagnostic Tests

Although detecting disease at an early stage in order to maximize treatment opportunities sounds logical, in practice it simply has not worked. Mammograms do not reduce the risk of dying from breast cancer.[111] Prostate cancer screening has not reduced the death rate from prostate cancer.[112] [113] Bypass surgery does not prevent fatal cardiovascular events.[114] [115] Millions of patients are being diagnosed with diseases they do not have, such as osteoporosis (see the chapter on women's health). And lots of doctors are prescribing drugs such as Tamoxifen and surgical procedures such as prophylactic mastectomy for disease prevention that have little or no positive effect.[116] It is understandable that more people are questioning whether or not to subject themselves to what Dr. John McDougall calls "The Medical Mill."

I do think it is important for everyone to make up their own mind about this issue. My life's work is dedicated to teaching people to think for themselves and to make informed decisions based on scientific data, not just telling people what to do. But the scientific evidence is clear; the money and resources we are spending on diagnostic testing and treatment is not improving Americans' health by reducing the incidence or death rate from the major degenerative diseases. The only method proven to accomplish those objectives is dietary excellence™ (a Wellness Forum-style diet) and optimal habits.

A common response from people when I present this information at lectures is "What do you tell the people who just won't practice dietary excellence? Isn't it better for these people to have diagnostic tests?" I don't think so, since they do not reduce the risk of dying from the conditions they are designed to detect. I think we have to be clear with people about their options – take care of yourself properly or there are negative consequences.

What do financial planners tell clients who won't save money? What do teachers tell kids who won't do their homework? And what do athletic coaches tell athletes who won't work out?

There are some things in life for which there are no shortcuts, and health is one of them.

Children's Health and Nutrition

"Children have never been very good at listening to their elders, but they have never failed to imitate them."

James Baldwin

Most parents are very diligent about their children's friends, their language development, the schools they attend, their academic performance, and almost every aspect of their lives. Yet a commonly neglected area in most families is diet.

I am convinced there are a variety of reasons for this, these are a few of the most common:

- Lack of knowledge about proper nutrition
- Conflicting information about diet
- Peer pressure from other children
- Lack of control over what children eat when they are away from home
- Not wanting to make children feel "different"
- Thinking children will outgrow their poor habits
- Thinking children's habits are "not that bad" or "not any worse than anyone else's kids"
- Fear of children disliking their parents

There are probably a few I've missed, but almost every parent I have talked to about their child's poor eating habits has cited at least one or two of these reasons as an obstacle to change.

Children's eating habits are extremely important – as important as making sure that they learn to say please and thank you, do their homework, and return home on time. Your child's future quality of life depends on what he or she learns from you about the importance of proper nutrition. Your child is not going to outgrow his poor habits, and, if your child eats some version of the Standard American Diet, he is almost assured of experiencing health problems in the future. Just like not doing homework and excelling in school positively affect job prospects in the future, eating the right foods positively affects future health.

Poor Eating Habits Start Early

According to a study called the Feeding Infants and Toddler's Study,[117] commissioned by Gerber Products, children's bad eating habits begin very early in life. The eating habits of more than 3000 children between the ages of 4 months and two years of age were recorded by asking their parents or primary caregivers what they ate on a particular day.

Here are the results:

- Children 1-2 years old require about 950 calories per day. The study showed that the average calorie intake of children in that age range was 1220 calories per day, 30% more than what is required. For children in the 7 to 11-month age range, the excess was 20%. Children are learning to overeat at a very early age.
- 1/3 of the children under 2 years old had no fruit or vegetables on the day of the survey.
- For those that did have a vegetable, French fries were the most common for children 15 months and older.
- 9% of children 9-11 months of age ate French fries at least once per day. For children 19 months to 2 years old, more than 20% had fries daily.
- 7% of the children 9 to 11 months old ate hot dogs, sausage and bacon daily, while 25% in the older age group ate these foods daily.
- Over 60% of the one-year olds had dessert or candy at least once per day and 16% ate a salty snack daily. By 19 months old, the percentages were 70% for dessert and candy and 27% for salty snacks.
- 40% of children 15 months and up had a sugary fruit drink each day, and 10% were already consuming soft drinks daily.
- 29% of infants were eating solid food before the age of 4 months
- 17% drank juice before the age of 6 months
- 20% were drinking cow's milk before the age of 12 months

These children will most likely continue these eating habits throughout the rest of their childhood, encouraged by advertising on television, offerings in the school cafeteria, and, in some cases, incorrect recommendations from health professionals.

Kids Also Need Exercise and Sleep

Fewer and fewer kids are getting enough physical activity; instead they are spending their time indoors watching television, playing on the computer, and texting their friends. Lack of physical activity not only promotes weight problems, but also leads to increased stress and anxiety, sleep disorders, lack of sunlight, and weakened bones (the biggest predictor of bone health in adults is physical activity in adolescence).

Kids are also sleep deprived. Their rooms are set up as multi-media playgrounds with televisions, computers and telephones and they are often using these "toys" long after bedtime. Many children are over-obligated, playing on multiple sports teams and participating in too many activities. This places enormous stress on families, as parents taxi kids to several activities daily while trying to work full-time jobs and manage a household. The resulting lack of sleep and downtime has an adverse effect on mood, can contribute to the development of depression, and can result in inability to concentrate and learn in school. It doesn't help the parents' health status much either.

Helping our kids get healthier involves improving their diets, making sure they get adequate exercise, and enough sleep every night.

Our Children Have Become
Unhealthy and Overweight

Due to their poor diets and lack of exercise, American children are suffering from an unprecedented number of physical problems:

- Children as young as three years of age have elevated c-reactive protein levels, a marker for inflammation[118]
- Children as young as six have thickening of the artery walls similar to 45-year olds[119]
- The fastest growing population of overweight people in the country is children. More than 9 million children between the ages of 6 and 19 are overweight;[120] 11% of infants between the ages of 6 and 23 months are overweight.[121]
- The American Academy of Family Physicians states that hypertension among children is increasing and now recommends that children be checked for it starting at the age of three.[122]
- Children are developing diseases formerly associated with older people such as type two diabetes and autoimmune diseases

Decision Time

As a parent, you often intervene with your child in matters such as a behavior pattern that you find inappropriate, or when academic performance begins to slide. It is just as important to intervene when your child's eating habits are unhealthy. This means taking charge of your household and making better decisions about food. This involves educating yourself about proper nutrition and becoming proactive with other family members, school officials, your child's friends and their parents, and everyone who provides him with food.

Will this be difficult? Absolutely! However, most people will do what is necessary if they have a strong reason. And the reason to do this is that your child's life may depend on it.

The Health Promoting Diet For Kids

The best diet for children is the same one that I recommend for adults:
- Plant-based – 90% (or more) of calories from fruits, vegetables, whole grains, legumes, nuts and seeds
- A maximum of 10% of calories from animal foods (which are optional)
- Eliminate dairy foods
- Low-fat – a maximum of 15% of calories from fat (except for children under the age of two; they require more fat)
- Reduced intake of minimally processed foods
- Eliminate daily consumption of refined foods
- Water as the first choice beverage
- Differentiate between food and a treat.

Age Appropriate Recommendations

Feeding Your Baby

Breast feeding is the best choice for infants, as this was what Mother Nature intended. Studies show that breast-fed babies are healthier, have stronger immune systems, better cognitive development, decreased incidence of speech and behavioral difficulties, and decreased risk of infections, diabetes, asthma, heart disease, obesity, multiple sclerosis, allergies, Ulcerative Colitis, Crohn's Disease and many other conditions throughout life.

While breastfeeding, it is important to pay attention to your diet, as this affects the health of your baby. First, you will need to consume about 20% more calories than you did prior to your pregnancy in order to meet the nutritional demands of your baby. Of course, you will want to stay away from caffeine, alcohol and other negative foods, as these are not good for your infant.

If you opt to eat a vegetarian diet while nursing, you should take a vitamin B12 supplement in order to insure your baby's healthy development. Although an adult's need for B12 is much lower than a baby's, and adults store the vitamin making deficiency unlikely, the demands of nursing require more B12.

Remember that whatever a nursing mom consumes, the baby ultimately consumes too. Eating a diet rich in whole, natural foods is the best way to meet your child's nutritional needs, and even to "program" his taste buds to want healthier foods when it is time to introduce solids.

If you decide for any reason not to nurse your baby, you'll be forced to make the best of essentially bad choices. Children who consume cow's milk have a much higher risk of developing juvenile diabetes.[123] [124] [125]
Cow's milk and soy milk formulas are not nutritionally identical to human breast milk. There is less risk associated with consuming organic soy formulas than cow's milk, perhaps making it the better of the less optimal options.

The superiority of human breast milk cannot be over-emphasized. So much so that Dr. John McDougall says that if he were Surgeon General, he would make formula available only by prescription.

Introducing Solids

Sometime between the ages of 4 and 6 months, it will be time to introduce foods other than breast milk or formula. At 4 months, a baby is generally not ready for solid food, as the swallowing reflex is not adequately developed. Juices, vegetable broth and applesauce in small amounts, however, are well tolerated.

At 6 months, babies are usually ready for a limited amount of solid food. It is important to add foods to the diet one at a time, so that food allergies can be identified. If your child doesn't like a particular food, serve it several times before giving up, as often repeated exposure results in acceptance of foods.

Try not to let your likes and dislikes influence your baby's food choices. Many parents assume that babies won't like foods because *they* don't like them and are quite surprised to find out that babies *do* like foods like beets and cabbage if they are repeatedly offered.

One of the easiest and most economical ways to provide the best nutrition is by making your own baby food at home. This can be done by placing fruits and vegetables with the skins removed, either cooked or raw, in a food processor or blender until pureed.

Purchasing Commercial Baby Food

Busy schedules dictate that you are not always going to be able to make your own baby food, so you will need to purchase some prepared foods at the store. Read labels carefully in order to avoid added sweeteners and other negative ingredients.

When to Introduce Foods

4-6 months:
    small amounts of fruit and vegetable juice
    applesauce
    vegetable broth

6-8 months:
- water
- fresh vegetables , mashed, such as avocado
- cooked vegetables, mashed, such as sweet potatoes, carrots, winter squash and peas
- fresh fruits, such as bananas and peaches, mashed

- gluten-free grains such as rice, millet, quinoa and buckwheat cereals, thinned with breast or formula
- soy milk and soy milk yogurt

<u>8-10 months</u>
- baked and mashed potatoes thinned with breast milk or formula
- well-cooked legumes, such as whole soybeans, garbanzo beans, kidney beans, lima beans, pinto beans, lentils and split peas, mashed or pureed
- fruit juices except citrus

<u>10-12 months</u>
- citrus juices and all other fruits
- thinned nut butters (use water, breast or soy milk)
- pasta, chopped small
- whole-grain bread
- gluten grains such as oats, rye and barley
- corn
- other soy foods such as tofu
- ground nuts and seeds
- organic poultry and meat

<u>1 year and older</u>
- other organic animal foods (optional)
- honey
- wild caught fish (optional)

Food Preparation for Babies

Grains
Brown rice, millet, barley, bread and cereals, oats

Grind up in a food mill or food processor. Cook 3 parts water to 1 part grain until food has a pasty consistency. Add soy milk or expressed breast milk.

Legumes
Soybeans, lentils, split peas, garbanzo beans, kidney beans, pinto beans

Legumes should be cooked in 3-4 parts water and then pureed or mashed. Soaking and cooking legumes well makes them much easier for a baby to digest.

Vegetables
Cut into thin slices and steam. Puree in a food processor or serve in small chunks.

Nuts and seeds
Process in a food processor until a buttery consistency. Mix with grains or rice, or for a more mature baby, roll into balls. Consume immediately, as this food does not keep well.

Dried fruits
For small babies, pulse in a food processor. Dried, pureed fruits can be added to a grain mixture, or eaten raw.

Fresh fruit
Mash with a fork or puree through a blender or food processor. Small pieces of fruit can be given to older babies to be eaten as finger food.

Tofu
Blend with fruit or vegetables in a blender or food processor.

Fruit Juices

Be careful when purchasing fruit juices, as most commercial baby juices have added sugar. Either juice fruits and vegetables yourself at home, or purchase juices that are labeled "not from concentrate" at a store. Limit the consumption of juices, and make sure your baby is learning to drink small amounts of water daily.

Variety and Allergies

If you want your child to eat a wide variety of foods, you must introduce him to lots of different foods early in life. Studies show that familiarity with foods is the strongest factor in food selection for toddlers, even more significant than the sweetness of foods. Also, the tendency to develop food allergies is substantially reduced if foods are not over-consumed. Some common signs of an allergy to food include:

- vomiting
- itchy skin
- swelling of the lips, throat, tongue, face and head
- rashes
- difficulty breathing
- behavioral changes
- congestion
- dark circles under the eyes

If you suspect that a food is causing a problem, eliminate it from the diet for several days, and then reintroduce it. If the symptoms disappear within a few days of elimination and reappear after reintroduction, you probably have identified a food your baby does not tolerate well.

Commonly Asked Questions About Babies

How much fat should a baby consume?
50% of the calories from human breast milk are from fat. Until children are one year of age, they should consume 50% of calories from fat; 30% until they are two years old; then a maximum of 15% of calories from fat thereafter.

How much food should a baby consume?
1-4 tablespoons is appropriate for 6-9 month-olds; for 9-12 month-old babies, 3-6 tablespoons of food will be consumed at each meal or snack. There are no hard and fast rules about how much food your baby should eat – every baby is different and appetites can vary from day to day.

Can vegetarian babies be assured of getting enough protein and other nutrients?
Absolutely. You will need to pay attention to making sure that there are adequate calories and fat in the diet. Vegetarian foods tend to be high in fiber, which can be very filling for a baby or toddler and can result in reduced consumption of calories. Nut butters and foods like avocadoes and tofu should be included because they contain more concentrated calories and fat.

B12 supplementation is advisable for vegan babies. B12 is available in liquid form and can be administered with a dropper or in powdered form which can be sprinkled on food.

How much protein do babies need?
People are generally more concerned about this issue than they need to be. Protein needs for humans are quite small; human breast milk contains only 6% of calories from protein. A diet that provides enough calories daily will provide enough protein.

How important is it to purchase organic plant foods?
Babies eat more fruits, vegetables, juices, and other potentially pesticide-containing foods as a percentage of weight than the average adult does. And, their gastrointestinal systems are more permeable, making it easier to absorb toxins. Therefore, to the extent that you are financially able, purchase organic produce.

When should a baby start drinking water?
Introducing water at an early age is the best way to insure that your child will develop the habit of drinking water. It is also important that your child not consume lots of juices and other flavored beverages. Research shows that consuming calories in beverages does not result in reduced consumption of calories from food; this can contribute to weight gain and obesity during childhood.

Water should be filtered since tap water contains chemicals such as chlorine.

Make sure that babies do not consume water immediately before eating, as it may suppress their appetites.

Nutrition for Toddlers

Your toddler should be eating what the rest of the family is consuming at mealtime, with the exception of foods to which the child has a confirmed allergy.

Be careful about the tendency to over-feed. With all good intentions, many parents feel that children should learn not to waste food and insist that they clean their plates. But learning how to avoid waste should not involve overeating. Overeating is a bad habit to develop and a difficult one to break.

The best way to teach your child not to waste food is to serve small portions and make seconds available if your child wants them.

This is the time for teaching your child some healthy eating habits. Children need to learn to eat slowly and chew their food well, since chewing is the first step in proper digestion. This is also a good time to stress talking only when the mouth is empty.

Although it isn't always easy, I recommend that families eat meals together. Research shows that children who eat with their families eat healthier foods, and mealtime provides a great opportunity for sharing and conversation.

It is not unusual for toddlers to reject foods, even some that they previously seemed to love, as a way of asserting themselves. This is a phase and will pass (thank God!). The best way to handle such challenges is to avoid making them an issue or a contest of wills. Do not force your child to eat if he or she does not want to. Simply remove the uneaten food from the table and wait until the next meal.

Do not make the mistake of turning your kitchen into a cafeteria. Many parents become panicked when their children do not eat for a day or two, and in an effort to get them to eat, begin to offer other options, including sweet treats, as an inducement to eat. There are two major problems with this approach. First, you will be sending the very clear message that your toddler is in charge. This will come back to haunt you, not only in the area of food consumption, but also in other areas as well.

Second, you will set a dangerous precedent – your child will believe that refusal to eat nutritious foods will result in access to foods of his choosing, including junk foods.

Most children have a healthy sense of self-preservation. In other words, they will not let themselves starve. A few skipped meals in order to establish some ground rules about dinnertime will not hurt your child, and, when he gets hungry enough, he will eat the nutritious fare you serve. Of course, if refusal to eat goes on for a long time, or you think there are health issues causing your child not to have an appetite, consult with your pediatrician immediately.

From a very early age, children should be taught the concept of eating smaller amounts of food 5-6 times throughout the day, rather than eating 3 large meals.

Commonly Asked Questions About Toddlers

Does my child need vitamins?

If your toddler is eating a well-structured diet that includes a wide variety of fruits, vegetables and grains, vitamin supplementation is not necessary, with the exception of vitamin B12.

Should I allow my toddler to eat sweets?

This is a personal decision. The reality is that sooner or later, your child is going to be introduced to candy, cookies and other unhealthy foods. The goal is to teach your child how to eat an optimal diet, and to differentiate between food and a treat. Too much restriction may backfire, as your child may decide that anything that is that "bad" must indeed be wonderful and worth obtaining at any cost!

Birthday parties and other special occasions are the most likely places for your child to be served cakes, cookies, etc. Small amounts of these foods, on special days, are okay. However, you must be careful to not allow this type of food to creep into your child's diet on a regular basis. This may mean talking with day care workers, grandparents, and others and making your wishes known, in addition to carefully controlling the food you allow in your own home

What do I do if my child continually asks for sweets?

It is not unusual for children to ask for more refined and processed foods once they are exposed to them. It is best to maintain your resolve to keep these foods out of your home and to maintain their status as treats. Therefore when your child asks for something sweet, offer dried or fresh fruit, natural cereals, or other foods that are regularly a part of your household diet. If your child declines, you can assume that she is not really hungry.

Sometimes my child is not hungry. Is this normal?

Absolutely. The appetite of a toddler varies from day to day. Also, children grow more slowly between the ages of 1 and 3, so it is normal for food consumption to be reduced somewhat. Another factor is that children often do not feel like eating when they are teething.

Don't try to get your child to eat if he really is not hungry. However, if the child refuses to eat for a long period of time, or you feel something is wrong, consult with your pediatrician immediately.

My child goes to day care. What do I do about the food served there?

Schedule a visit with the Director or owner of the center your child attends and inquire about the food that is offered to children. If it not acceptable, explain that you will be providing the food to serve your child while at daycare.

If you encounter resistance, find another center. Remember you are the client and you have the right to be just as concerned about the food that your child eats as you are about the children your child spends time with and the activities she is engaged in while at daycare.

If you are lucky, the director may be interested in knowing more about healthy eating and your lifestyle, and be open to changing the food that is served in the center. If so, recommend Wellness Forum programming in order for the staff to learn more about optimal diets.

My toddler has not been eating healthy foods, and I want to change that. What if he doesn't like them?

It is normal for kids to reject healthier foods if they are used to eating sweets and junk foods. You may get more cooperation by offering new foods in conjunction with familiar ones. For example, you might include a new vegetable in a familiar soup or casserole. It can take several exposures to a food over a period of time before your child will eat it.

Remember that your child's eating habits were developed over a period of time, and they will usually not change overnight. Be patient and stick with it. Refusing to eat is your child's way of testing your resolve. If you give in and bring back the junk food, it will be even more difficult to make changes in the future because your child will know that refusal to eat results in getting the foods he wants. When things get difficult, remember how important nutrition is for your child's future.

Nutrition for Preschoolers

By the time your child is 3 years old, you can begin to have conversations about the importance of good nutrition, just as you have conversations about manners and other topics. Teaching your children a value system about food and nutrition is important and can be done at a very early age. Children are interested in becoming "big and strong." They are also, at this age, interested in pleasing the adults in their life. Capitalize on this!

Preschoolers are old enough to understand the difference between healthy foods and junk foods, if you take the time to explain it to them. This should be an ongoing process, as you make healthy eating part of your family's "culture."

The Television is Not Your Friend!

Limiting television viewing is better for children and can help you in promoting a healthier diet. The television is not a very good companion or babysitter for children of any age, and much of the content is inappropriate for kids. The added problem is that television programming includes a constant barrage of ads from food manufacturers and fast food outlets, all designed to make your child want their products. According to the Center for Science in the Public Interest (CSPI) in Washington, D.C., fast food and sugary cereals are the most commonly advertised foods on television. [126] Food companies spend hundreds of millions of dollars on advertising every year for a very good reason – it works!!!

Additionally, you must think about the impression that television shows make on young minds. The stars are often shown eating junk food, but they look beautiful and healthy. Very few are overweight. This sends the erroneous message that there are no negative consequences from eating these foods. But we all know better!

When Your Child Wants Fast Food

No matter how much you talk to your child and serve healthy foods, he will most likely ask for fast food. Here's a helpful tip for responding to your child's requests. Fast food companies have become adept at luring children into wanting their high-fat, processed fare by offering all kinds of non-food rewards, such as characters from the latest popular movie for children. Sometimes it is the reward that is motivating the desire to eat fast food, not the food itself.

Occasionally pack up a healthy picnic lunch or dinner and include a "prize" in it similar or identical to the one being offered by the local burger joint. Your child will associate healthful meals with rewards and it may reduce the number of requests to consume garbage!

Some fast food companies are offering healthier fare (baked potatoes can be ordered without the usual toppings, salads without cheese, etc.); hopefully this trend will continue.

Getting Cooperation

This is a good time to allow your child to participate in meal preparation. In addition to providing some quality time for you to be together, this is an opportunity to relate nutritional information about foods you've chosen while you're fixing them, rather than at the dinner table, where the conversation shouldn't always revolve around a discussion of what's served.

Take children to the grocery store with you. Allow them to choose new foods to try. For example, suggest that your child pick a new fruit or vegetable that he finds interesting. Or present two healthy cereals and let your child choose which one to buy. Ask your children to help you fill your cart with different colored foods – ask them to see how many different ones they can find. Make it fun. Participation leads to cooperation.

Lead by Example

Leading by example is most important. By now, your child is keenly aware of everything you do, and is very interested in imitating you. This is an extremely important time for *showing* your child the importance of good eating in addition to talking about it.

Practice "Health by Deception"

If you have made the decision to change the family's eating habits, one way to lessen resistance is to start with healthy foods that taste familiar. Some ideas might be pizza without cheese on a whole grain crust, vegetable soup without chicken, and chili using ground tempeh instead of meat. It's sometimes best not to draw unneeded attention to the healthier offerings. You don't need to announce that there is tofu in the casserole the next time you serve lasagna. You might be surprised at how well some of these foods are received. Ignorance can be bliss.

What About Desserts?

I have always advised against dessert becoming a part of every meal. This encourages too much consumption of unhealthy foods, and it often positions dessert as a reward for eating dinner. A child should consume dinner because he is hungry, not due to the promise of something sweet as a reward. Dessert at every meal can send a negative message – dessert is "good", while the foods served for dinner are less than desirable, and therefore a reward is due for eating them.

If you serve anything after a meal, fruit is the best option. Save cake and cookies for birthday parties and other special occasions; remember that these foods are treats.

Commonly Asked Questions About Preschoolers

My child often does not eat at mealtime. Is there a problem?

There are several reasons why a child may not eat at mealtime. One is not being hungry. Take a look at when your child is eating. Too much water, snacks eaten too close to dinner time, or too many high-fiber foods can suppress the appetite.

Children sometimes do not eat because they are too tired to eat. The need for sleep always supersedes the need for food. Your child may need more sleep at night or a longer nap.

I am getting a lot of resistance to new foods. What should I do?

This can be difficult, but you are going to have to make a firm commitment to stick with your plan regardless of the resistance you get from your child. Just as you will not allow a teenager to stay out all night, no matter how unpopular your decision, you must decide that your child's health is important and that you will be making the decisions about what he eats. It is very important for parents to be in charge.

Set a date by which there will be no more "bad" food in your house. If these foods are not available they will not be consumed. Stick with your decision.

Begin offering a choice between only healthy alternatives. For example, you might present an apple and a banana as snack options. If your child chooses neither, then you can assume he is not hungry. If your child suggests a candy bar instead, you can respond by saying "We don't have any candy bars here – we only have fruit for snacks. Now, would you like a banana or an apple?"

If you are consistent, eventually, your child will figure out that candy is no longer an option for a snack and begin to choose from your healthier options. If you give in, you will have to repeat the process again and again until your child knows that the rules have changed permanently. Each time the process will become more difficult, since your child will operate under the assumption that enough resistance will bring back the foods he wants.

At dinnertime, serve healthy meals. Although you will want to show some consideration for likes and dislikes (if your child hates kidney beans, for example, you can avoid those and serve other types of beans instead), serve a healthy meal and let your child decide whether or not to eat. If your child does not choose to eat, don't force him or her. However, if the child is hungry later and asks for food, offer the leftover dinner. If he still refuses, that's okay. Do not offer another option. You do not want to give your child the idea that refusing to eat dinner is a way to get the foods he wants to eat. Remember, you are in charge!

School-Aged Children

Once children begin to attend school, peer pressure becomes a factor. Children want to fit in with their friends and classmates, and they are likely at this time to take notice of the fact that their diet is "different." Additionally, their desire for more independence may make maintaining your healthy lifestyle challenging.

It is very important to continually communicate with your child and explain the reasons why you choose the foods you choose. You are a very important role model for your child – make sure you are practicing healthy habits too. Parents are powerful influences – you can make a bigger difference than you think by talking about and demonstrating your values about nutrition and health.

It is also very important to learn to compromise. Allowing cookies or other treats on special occasions is reasonable and appropriate. Always withholding these foods can be counterproductive.

The School Cafeteria

Some of the worst food your child eats is in the school cafeteria. The school lunch program is administered by the USDA, an agency burdened with conflicts of interest, as you learned earlier.

Congress created the National School Lunch Program to "safeguard the health and well being of the nation's children and to encourage the domestic consumption of nutritious agricultural commodities." Unfortunately, there is an inherent conflict in trying to accomplish both of these goals through the school lunch program – promotion of agricultural commodities may not be best for our children's health.

Prior to allowing a child to purchase lunch at school, parents should visit the school cafeteria during lunchtime to find out what is being served. While some schools are offering healthier fare, these are unfortunately exceptions rather than the rule.

One of the reasons why school lunches are so unhealthy is that the USDA gives schools commodities it buys from farmers in order to provide price support for agricultural products. These commodity foods constitute as much as 20% of the food served and include butter, cheddar cheese, ground beef, lunch meat, ham, eggs, salted canned vegetables, and canned fruit in heavy syrup.

As if this isn't bad enough, many school cafeterias also contract out food service to fast food restaurants.

If your child's school does not offer healthy foods, the best option is to pack your child's lunch as often as possible. If your child loves the food offered in the cafeteria (this is entirely possible, based on the fact that it's full of fat and sugar), a compromise might be necessary. Most schools publish in advance the menus for the week. Allow your child to pick one day per week to buy a school lunch if she brings lunch the rest of the week.

Allowing your child to have some input into what goes into his lunch can help you to gain some cooperation too. Here are some suggestions:

Sandwiches
Breads:
> Pita bread
> Wholegrain bread
> Whole grain bagels

Tortillas (flat like a quesadilla or rolled)
Wholegrain English Muffins
Whole Grain Sandwich style bun

Fillings:
Refried Beans with red bell pepper or cucumber and salsa
Nut butter and spreadable fruit
Nut butter and strawberry, apple or banana slices
Nut butter and grated carrots
Nut butter with raisins or dried cherries
Fat-free hummus, shredded carrots and celery
Fat-free hummus on whole wheat bread
Fat-free hummus with tomatoes, cucumber and lettuce
Hummus mixed with grated carrots and spinach or other
lettuce
Leftover rice with lettuce, tomatoes and salad dressing in
a wrap
Tofu egg salad with lettuce
Make a pizza quesadilla with pizza toppings (sauce, tofu
pepperoni, pinch of rice or soy cheese or veggie with olives,
mushrooms, onions, spinach, squash, eggplant, etc)
Veggie burger with mustard, ketchup, pickles, tomatoes,
onion, etc
Vegetarian chili

Asian theme:
Sobo noodles with peanut sauce (available in health foods
stores)
Sugar Snap Peas
Pear
Fortune cookie

Mexican theme:
Taco Salad #1
Lettuce topped with tempeh taco filling (Wellness Forum
Taco Taco mix is terrific and is good hot or cold!) tomatoes,
onions, olives, salsa, vegan sour cream, guacamole

Taco Salad #2
Substitute black beans and rice for taco filling

Mediterranean theme:
 Fat-free hummus topped with spinach on a tortilla
 Cherry tomatoes
 Soy Yogurt

Some prep is required for these dishes but they keep for several days:
(recipes in the Wellness Forum's Big and Healthy Cookbook)
 Mock "Egg" salad
 Mock "Chicken" Salad
 Mock "Tuna" Salad
 Peanut noodles
 Wellness Forum Brown Rice Vegetable Soup with mushrooms, miso and spinach

Potatoes:
 ½ baked potato topped with just about anything...soup, salsa, Wellness Forum "Cheese" sauce or vegetable chili
 ½ sweet potato topped with cinnamon
 Healthy French-fries for occasional treat (these can be purchased in the frozen foods section of the health food store, or you can make at home in the oven with oil-free dressing)

Pasta:
 Different macaroni shapes topped with:
  Wellness Forum Cheese sauce
  Red sauce and vegetables
  Vegetarian chili
  Any other hearty soup, like black bean, potato

Brown rice, quinoa or couscous:
 Pair with any vegetables (fresh, steamed or frozen) and/or beans and add any of the following:
 Salsa
 Bragg's Liquid Aminos
 Spaghetti sauce
 Salad Dressing (fat-free)
 Cooked potatoes (redskin or Yukon gold hold shape best)
 Sprouts (grow them yourself)
 Tofu cubes
 Dried fruit

Any dried soup mix, Wellness Forum or others like Dr. McDougall Soups

Some suggested combinations
Salsa, corn, black beans and sprouts
Spaghetti sauce, peas or steamed eggplant
Spinach, garbanzo beans with fat-free dressing
Potatoes, raisins and pine nuts, sprinkled with curry powder
Lima beans, corn, peas and Braggs
Potatoes, green beans and chopped cooked onions
Stewed tomatoes, kidney beans sprinkled with chili powder
Salad, split peas, dressing and sprouts
Steamed broccoli, cauliflower, walnuts, sprinkled with dry onion soup
Wellness Forum cheese sauce mixed with Wellness Forum What a tomato soup, tofu cubes

Getting Cooperation

As soon as your child can read, you can involve him in the process of selecting foods. Turn grocery shopping into a game. Ask your children to find a cereal that does not contain sugar, or a spaghetti sauce without oil. Allow them to choose new fruits and vegetables.

Hand your child a vegetarian cookbook and ask him to pick out a recipe to try. Any activity that gets children involved in the process will help them to make better choices willingly.

Controlling When and
How Much Food is Consumed

Even parents who stock only healthy foods in the house can run into problems with overeating or eating at inappropriate times, such as 15 minutes before dinner time or late at night. Particularly when children are younger, it is important to control not only what, but how much and when food is eaten.

When your children come home from school, offer a snack of cut-up fruit or veggies and dip. Put the food on a plate and insist

144

that the child eat at a kitchen or dining room table. You can prepare food in advance if your child is with a babysitter after school, and insist on the same protocol. Food consumption should be restricted to certain areas of the house such as the kitchen and the dining room and eating generally should not accompany other activities, particularly television watching, except on special occasions. Unlimited amounts of food consumed while wandering throughout the house often leads to overeating and "mindless eating."

Nutrition for Adolescents

The reality is that as children get older, they spend less time at home, which means that you will have less control over the food they eat.

If your children have been brought up on a healthy diet and understand the reasons why you have made the choices you have made in this area, you will have a foundation upon which to continue your discussions about health and nutrition. Keep in mind that it is normal for even healthy eaters to want to eat junk food, and to want to fit in with their friends. You can almost be assured that your teen is going to eat some fast food and junk at least some of the time. If most of what they eat is healthy, however, you should not make an issue out of the food that isn't.

If you are just beginning to change the family's diet, involve your teenagers in the process. Invite them to participate in Wellness Forum courses with you, and provide them with DVD's and other materials that can assist them in arriving at the right conclusions about nutrition and health. *Be patient!*

Sometimes adolescents become more interested in healthier dietary habits because they are interested in the effects of diet on the environment and in animal rights issues. Most adolescents think they are invincible, and preventing heart disease and cancer does not seem relevant to them. The film *Diet for a New America* offers a great discussion of health that includes information about the environmental impact of a diet based on animal foods. Mercy For Animals is a non-profit organization that conducts undercover investigations of factory farms and advocates for elimination of these operations (www.mercyforanimals.org). Exposing teens to these resources may do more to convince them to change their diets than talking about personal health. Teenagers are interested in the appearance, weight and in sports performance, so information on the relationship between diet and these issues can be very convincing.

While you can't control what your teenagers eat away from home, you *can* still control the food that is available in the house. You do not have to purchase soft drinks, doughnuts and potato chips, or serve unhealthy foods at mealtime. Of course there will be exceptions, but maintain your resolve to promote the health of your child with the same diligence you exercise in monitoring his friends, his grades, and other aspects of his life.

A word of encouragement – I have talked to many parents who have felt that their attempts to encourage healthy eating have been for naught, only to find later on that it did a lot more good than they previously thought. Kids remember the way they were brought up and often, after they spread their wings and experiment on their own, come back to the ways of life they learned at home. Be consistent and set a good example, and you *will* make a difference.

Setting an Example

The most important thing parents can do to influence their children's lifestyle habits is to eat an excellent diet themselves, and to exercise on a regular basis. Leading by example has been proven to be a powerful influence on behavior for both kids and adults.

Do not underestimate the power of your behavior in determining the choices your children will make.

Making Healthy Habits Part of
Your Family's Culture

It will take time for your kids to understand that part of your family's value system includes the consumption of healthy foods and practicing healthy habits. But it takes time to teach your children everything else as well. Think about it. When your child reached the age of two, did you sit down for a one-time conversation during which you instructed him about the importance of saying "please" and "thank you," and sitting quietly while adults were talking and he just complied from that day forward? No – teaching these values required constant instruction and reinforcement until one day your child had become, for the most part, polite.

The same will be true about teaching your child about healthy eating. While you do not want to lecture and have every meal revolve around a discussion about why you are eating the way you do, you do want to engage in regular, age-appropriate conversation about the issue. Over time, your child will begin to understand why you are making some of the choices you are and gradually she will "buy in."

Common Situations for Families

My child doesn't like vegetables. What should I do?
Continue serving them, and experiment with various ways of preparing them. For example, your child may not like cooked carrots, but will eat them raw. Or, you may find that providing chopped vegetables with fat-free hummus promotes more vegetable eating. Serve vegetables first when children are hungriest and other meal items later.

"Health by deception" is also effective. In other words, "package" foods your child doesn't like in foods that are generally well-accepted. You can add small amounts of peas and corn to noodle soup, for example. Or combine small portions of vegetables in mashed potatoes. Pureeing beans in vegetable broth to use as a base for soup disguises the beans.

Continue to present vegetables as a staple of the diet, and do not offer to replace them with other foods. It can take a long time, but tastes can and do change.

My children often visit their grandparents and they insist on feeding them fried chicken and other unhealthy foods.
This is a difficult issue. But you must remember that you are the parent. Do not allow grandparents and other well-meaning

147

relatives and friends to "love your children to death" by feeding them unhealthy foods. Explain your views on proper nutrition and what you expect when your children are in their care. Compromising a little can help. For example, one unhealthy meal may be allowed if the rest of the food is according to plan. And, grandparents like to spoil children with candy and ice cream treats. Occasionally, this is all right. But it cannot and should not become an important part of the diet every time your children are with relatives.

Offer to provide food while your child is visiting his grandparents. Sometimes grandparents don't know what to serve in place of unhealthy foods.

Suggest that your child's grandparents read this book, or take Wellness Forum courses in order to understand why you have made the decisions you have made about food and health.

My parents/in-laws insist that a vegetarian diet is not appropriate or safe for my children.
It is normal for people to be concerned about the health and welfare of their grandchildren. However, a vegetarian or near-vegetarian diet is very safe and healthful – in fact – much safer than the Standard American Diet that most children eat!

Suggest that your family members read *The China Study* and take Wellness Forum courses. Often third-party information is more convincing than information from family members.

My child is a picky eater.
Some children are picky eaters because they have had little exposure to a variety of foods. Others are picky hoping that refusal to eat healthy foods will force you to give them what they want.

Serve a variety of healthy foods consistently and your child will learn to eat them. Of course, there are going to be some foods your child doesn't like. This is normal and a child should not be forced to eat scalloped potatoes if she genuinely doesn't like them. But there is a difference between acknowledging normal likes and dislikes and allowing your child to live on junk or very few foods for an extended period of time because he refuses to eat the right foods.. Remember, you are the parent!

My child only wants to eat unhealthy foods.
Stop providing these foods, and cut off the supply of these foods from other sources. When a parent states that her child only wants to eat Fruit Loops and potato chips, a logical question is "where's the child getting the food?" Most 6-year olds do not go grocery shopping, which means adults are responsible for providing the food. STOP!

My child often doesn't finish his dinner.
There are 2 reasons why a child may not finish a meal. The portions may be too big. If this is the case, cut back on the amount of food you serve and allow your child to ask for seconds if necessary.

The other reason is the child is making a statement about the food. He would rather have something else to eat. If this is the reason, do not force the child to eat or turn mealtime into a nightmare. Simply remove the plate from the table and save it for later in the event that the child indicates that he is hungry. Do not be manipulated into serving different or unhealthy foods, or providing desserts and sweets later. A child will not be harmed by going to bed hungry a few times and will soon learn to eat the dinner that is served.

What should I do when my child plays at other children's houses?
Again, remember who is in charge of your child's welfare and health. Talk with the parent who is home supervising the play activities and explain your family's eating habits. Offer to provide snacks or meals for the children yourself.

Some compromise may be necessary in order to keep your child from being isolated, but under no circumstances should your child be able to consume large amounts of unhealthy food at other people's houses on a regular basis.

This is an analogy that might help you. If your child was allergic to a particular food, you would make sure that everyone feeding your child would know about that so as to avoid disaster. You would certainly make sure that your child was aware of the food allergy and the consequences of consuming that food. Eating junk is no different – you can make your child aware of the consequences and instill in her a desire to take proper care of herself, and you can insist that those who are entrusted with her care show the same respect.

My former spouse doesn't agree that healthy foods are important.
This is a common form of disagreement between divorced parents, and how to handle it varies depending on your relationship with your ex.

If you are on good terms, you should sit down to discuss this issue and arrive at a compromise that satisfies both of you, keeping the best interest of your child in mind.

If you are not on good terms, this might be a good opportunity to make the first move toward working together to do what is best for your children. Parents should always try to put their differences aside in order to take proper care of their children. This may mean "giving in" or a feeling of losing control, but your child's future is much more important than your ego. Providing your ex with written information (such as this book) about the benefits of this diet and the detrimental effects of your child's current diet can help. It is almost always better for your ex to learn about this diet from a third party, rather than insisting that he/she listen to you.

If negotiation is not a possibility, you will have to do the best you can by making sure that your child eats healthy food when he is with you. Without putting down the other parent, explain why you provide the foods you do and how important it is to pay attention to good health. If your child asks why they are allowed to eat certain foods at your ex's house, **do not say negative things about your ex!** Instead, say "Daddy/mommy doesn't know any better now but is doing the best he/she can."

Many people confuse food and love. Weekend parents, trying to gain favor with a child in the short amount of time they have, may think they are "buying influence" by providing unhealthy foods that are not available at the other parent's house. This issue also comes up with discipline – a weekend parent can be wary of disciplining a child, thinking the child won't like him or her if they are forced to behave in a certain way.

The reverse is actually true, however. The best way to show love to your child is to provide healthy foods, and to insist on proper behavior and responsibility in a loving environment. Your child innately knows this, even though it may seem that she gravitates to the parent that is the most permissive. Many parents find that in the process of trying to make their child "like" them, that they lose the respect of the child and have to work to regain it.

With patience and the right approach, children can come around. Often they start asking for healthy foods. They may start to notice the difference in how they feel while on a junk food diet at the other parent's house vs. at yours. They may notice differences in your health vs. your ex's.

And, there have been instances where an ex-spouse develops an interest in improving her diet by learning from her children. Miracles do happen!

My child has a weight problem. I don't want to make her feel self-conscious, but I want to motivate her to lose weight.
If your child is overweight, she is already very self-conscious, and ignoring the problem will not make it go away.

First, examine the reasons why your child is overweight. Are the portions you are serving at mealtime too large? Is your child eating junk food? Are you allowing too much snacking? Too many second helpings? Is your child sedentary?

Once you have assessed the reasons why your child has a weight problem, you can begin to change diet and exercise patterns, which should result in weight loss. You don't need to draw a lot of attention to what you are doing. Simply convert to a Wellness Forum-style diet immediately. Get the "bad" foods out of the house. Put less food on the dinner plate. Ask your child to join you for bike rides or walking. Studies consistently show that kids of active parents are significantly more likely to be active as adults than children of sedentary parents.

If your child's weight does not begin to change within a reasonable period of time, consult with your pediatrician or other health care professional to determine if there are other factors contributing to the problem.

My child is attending college and living in a dorm. How can he maintain a healthy diet when the food in the dorm is so bad?
College food service is getting a little better, with some colleges serving more vegetarian fare. Hopefully by the time your child leaves home to go to school, he will have learned how to pick the best alternatives in a cafeteria or restaurant setting.

Most college students are allowed to have a refrigerator and other appliances in their rooms. When you move your child into the dorm, locate the nearest store that sells fresh produce.

Provide "care packages" from home containing foods that may not be readily available near the university.

Since breakfast is such an important meal and healthy breakfast food can be hard to find in a dining hall, set up the dorm room to make Dr. Pam Popper's Healthy Breakfast Smoothie in the morning. Blenders and coffee grinders (for flax) don't take up much room.

What do we do at holiday times when we eat with family members that do not make healthy eating a priority?
It is highly unlikely that you are going to convince all of your relatives to prepare healthy food for your next holiday celebration. If some family members are approachable about changing the menu, then discuss it with them. If not, you are going to have to work around the "bad" food. In any case, it might be a good idea to make sure that those in charge of the food know how you and your children will be eating at your gathering.

One easy solution is to offer to bring part of the meal. Most hosts are appreciative of any help with food preparation, and this way you can make sure that there are some healthy selections available. Be sure to choose dishes that not only your children like, but that most others will like as well. Your children are obviously more likely to eat the foods you bring if you bring favorites. Also, you may make progress with the rest of the family by practicing "health by deception" – serving something absolutely delicious, but healthy, that they do not *know* is healthy!

Discuss the situation with your children in advance, reminding them that not everyone eats the way that you do, but emphasizing why you make the choices you make. Compromise can be an important part of surviving holiday celebrations. Allowing children to have a couple of their favorite things as a treat, while eating the healthier foods you bring, is one way to compromise. This should be talked about in advance of the holiday gathering in order to avoid conflict.

What do I do about Halloween?
Every year, shortly after Halloween, lots of children who have been healthy for months or years get sick. No wonder – many of them are on a steady daily diet of sugar following Beggar's Night.

Most parents will not take the unpopular stand of forbidding children to go out Trick-or-Treating. If your children are really young, however, you may be able to organize a Beggar's Night for them with a few other households whose philosophies are in line with yours. Most small children aren't up for visiting more than a few houses anyway, and this way you can control the treats they get.

If your children are too old to be restricted in this way, allow them to gather their candy, let them choose a few favorite pieces to eat for a day or two, and GET RID OF THE REST. Your child does not need to eat several hundred calories of sugar daily for weeks after Beggar's Night! (It probably isn't such a good idea for you to have it around either!)

My child wants to have other children over to play. What should I serve them?
When children visit your home, serve them the foods your children are accustomed to eating. Fruit, healthy cookies, veggies and dip, and frozen fruit juice treats are usually liked by all kids. You may get some of your child's friends interested in

healthy eating, and seeing their friends enjoying the foods you serve will reinforce the fact that healthy food tastes good.

Women's Health

I love educating women about optimal health. Women are often the decision makers in the household about nutrition and health. They are usually caregivers for spouses, children, parents, and others. When I convince women that The Wellness Forum's diet is the right way to eat, they will almost always influence other people to make positive dietary changes too.

I also love educating women because they are often victimized by unnecessary testing, false diagnoses, and over-treatment by the medical profession.

And last but not least, women tend to put the care of others first before themselves. While on the one hand this is admirable, the downside is that it often results in women not paying adequate attention to their own health. While taking care of everyone else, exercise, healthy eating, rest, and sleep often go by the wayside, and weight gain and health issues often develop.

When women practice dietary excellence™ and optimal habits, their appearance, weight, and overall health improve. But they also can set a great example for others they care about, particularly children. They can avoid common degenerative diseases that can be time consuming, expensive, and interfere with family life. And, they will have the energy needed not only to do all the things they want to do for themselves, but to care for children, parents, and others close to them.

This section of the book deals with issues of interest to most women; reproductive health, mammography and breast cancer, weight, menopause, and bone health.

Birth Control Pills and Cancer Risk

On July 29, 2005, the International Agency for Research on Cancer, a division of the World Health Organization, issued a press release stating that combined estrogen-progestin contraceptives are carcinogenic,[127] and concluded that the pills can increase the risk of breast, liver, and cervical cancer.

An article in the *New England Journal of Medicine* concluded that oral contraceptives increase the risk of breast cancer between 20 and 30%.[128]

Researchers at Oxford University found that the risk of cervical cancer was related to the length of time a woman spent on oral contraceptives.[129] Women who had used them for less than 5 years had a 10% increased risk, those who took them for 5-9 years had a 60% increased risk, and for those who used them for more than 10 years, there was a 120% increased risk. The risk was even higher in women who were both infected with the human papilloma virus (HPV) and took oral contraceptives.

Researchers reported at an American Heart Association meeting that long-term use of birth control pills was linked to increased plaque build-up in the neck and legs. They stated that for every 10 years a woman takes oral contraceptives, the risk of accumulating plaque in these arteries increased by 20-30%.[130]

In spite of this, doctors continue to prescribe oral contraceptives, even for young girls, for many conditions, including acne, PMS, and irregular periods.

There are better ways to deal with all of the health issues for which oral contraceptives are prescribed. For birth control, almost anything is better, but the best option in my opinion, is natural family planning, which has been shown to be just as effective as birth control pills. There are several methods, which include The Creighton Model FertilityCare System[131] and the Billings Ovulation Method.[132] The programs include instruction for women on how to track their cycles in order to determine when they are fertile

PMS symptoms like irregular periods, cramping and other discomfort, can be relieved by lowering estrogen levels through improved diet and exercise, and maintaining a lean body. Acne can almost always be resolved with dietary improvement and improving gastrointestinal health.

It is amazing to me that birth control pills continue to be widely prescribed, and I'm most disturbed by the number of young girls who are being advised to take them. Taking birth control pills increases their risk of cancer at a very early age, and prevents them from addressing the underlying causes of their health issues

158

Breast Health

Women are terrified of breast cancer, and for good reason. Once diagnosed, disfiguring surgery and toxic, debilitating treatments are often recommended. The risk of recurrence is high.

The medical profession, in conjunction with national health organizations like the American Cancer Society, promotes mammography screening. The message is that if found early, breast cancer is treatable and the best way to find it early is through mammography.

But mammography is highly unreliable. It tends to miss aggressive tumors that grow between screenings, while detecting small, benign tumors, such as carcinoma in situ, that are usually not cancers at all and are often referred to as "pseudo-cancers."

In spite of the fact that less than 2% of these "pseudo-cancers" will develop into a cancer requiring treatment, women diagnosed with them are advised to have lumpectomies, to receive radiation treatments, and to take drugs like Tamoxifen. This is over-treatment for a condition that is highly unlikely to be life threatening. Particularly troubling is how these women are classified as "cancer survivors." Almost all of them would be alive five years after diagnosis (the benchmark for survival for cancer patients) even with no treatment. This skews the survival statistics numbers, making it look like treatments for breast cancer are much more effective than they really are.

While mammography detects "pseudo-cancers" resulting in over-treatment, it does not reduce the risk of dying from real cases of breast cancer.

An article published in 2001 in the *Lancet*[133] reported the findings of a Cochrane Review that looked at the efficacy of mammograms for reducing breast cancer deaths. 500,000 women in the United States, Canada, Scotland and Sweden were included. The new report concluded that for every 2000 women who get mammograms over a 10-year period, only one would experience prolonged life, and 10 would endure unnecessary and potentially harmful procedures.

The Cochrane researchers further concluded that studies showing that mammograms reduce the risk of dying from breast cancer do not take into consideration the deaths related to breast cancer treatments, and stated, "there is no reliable evidence from large randomized trials to support screening mammography at any age."

A previous Cochrane Review reported no benefit for mammography at any age.

A study published online by the *British Medical Journal* [134] was conducted in Denmark, a great country for studying mammography outcomes. For the past 17 years, only about 20% of women in Denmark have been screened, leaving a large control group from which data can be gathered.

Two geographic areas were included in the study; Copenhagen, where screening was introduced in 1991, and Funen, where screening was introduced in 1997. Between 1997 and 2005, deaths from breast cancer dropped by 5% for women between the ages of 35 and 55 in both of these areas. For women between 55 and 74, the decline was 1% in mortality rate.

In the non-screened population in Denmark, the death rate from breast cancer declined by 6% for women between the ages of 35 and 55, and 2% for women between 55 and 74.

The researchers also observed that the diagnosis of carcinoma in situ doubled in the population of women who were screened and remained the same in the non-screened population, reinforcing the idea that mammography results in over-diagnosis of pseudo cancers.

Studies even show that mammography is contraindicated for women who carry the BRCA1 or BRCA2 gene mutation which predisposes them to a higher risk of developing breast cancer.[135] In one study, researchers concluded that mammography screening beginning at 25 to 29 years of age results in a higher risk of breast cancer due to increased lifetime radiation exposure, and that mammography may have a net harmful effect for these patients.

According to data from the University of Washington and Harvard, one of every two women who have mammograms regularly will have a false positive, and 20% will have an unnecessary biopsy.[136] For every $100 spent on mammograms, $33 is spent on addressing false positives.

Research conducted at Duke University Medical Center showed that the cost for unnecessary mammograms in women over 70 during the year 2000 alone was $460 million.[137]

The U.S. Preventive Services Task Force issued a report in 2009 concluding that the risks of mammograms for women between the ages of 40 and 50 outweighed any benefits; that women over 50 years of age should get mammograms every other year instead of annually; and that there was no justification for mammograms after the age of 74. The group also recommended against breast self-examination, since there was insufficient evidence that it is effective.[138]

I advise women not to get mammograms as a strategy for reducing their risk of dying from breast cancer. I am often challenged on this issue, often by women who know someone who was diagnosed with breast cancer through mammography and are convinced that the person is alive as a result. There *are* women who benefit from mammography, but the fact remains that *most* do not. Research shows that the risks outweigh the benefits for most women.

Reducing Your Risk of Breast Cancer

Women who are interested in reducing their risk of developing or dying from breast cancer should practice dietary excellence™ and optimal habits, as outlined in this book; it's the only strategy that has been proven to work. Most breast cancers are estrogen positive; a low-fat, plant-based diet helps to reduce estrogen levels.

Eliminating cow's milk and products made from cow's milk is important; cow's milk comes from pregnant cows and contains estrogen – even organic cow's milk contains estrogen.

Eating a high-fiber, plant-based diet helps too. Fiber assists in the elimination of waste products, including estrogen, which keeps it from being re-absorbed into the blood stream contributing to higher estrogen levels.

A low-fat plant-based diet contributes to weight loss. Adipose (fat) cells produce hormone-like compounds that function like estrogen. Losing weight can reduce your risk significantly.

And, exercise lowers estrogen levels. Lean, active women who eat a low-fat, plant-based diet have a much lower risk of developing breast cancer than their more overweight, carnivorous counterparts.

PMS and a Vegetarian Diet

Today, almost 10% of women in their teens and early 20's are suffering from severe menstrual cramps. The cause is uterine muscle contractions triggered by series 2 prostaglandins (PGE2), which are produced in the endometrial tissue from estrogen, progesterone, and dietary precursors such as animal foods.

A plant-based diet like the one recommended by The Wellness Forum is effective for reducing menstrual cramps and other PMS symptoms. The diet results in decreased estrogen level and increased production of sex-hormone binding globulin (SHBG), which inhibits the activity of estrogen. A plant-based diet also reduces products of inflammatory PGE2. Reduced estrogen and PGE2 levels, combined with higher SHBG levels causes a reduction in uterine contractions and therefore pain.

Women consuming a vegetarian, low-fat diet generally have lower body weight, and women with lower body weight tend to have higher concentrations of SHBG. The higher fiber content of a plant-based diet helps to eliminate estrogen through the feces, preventing it from being re-absorbed though the intestinal walls and into the blood stream.

Dr. Neal Barnard has conducted research confirming this phenomenon. Patients consuming a low-fat vegetarian diet experienced a 19% increase in SHBG levels, and the duration of

PMS symptoms including behavioral changes and water retention were significantly reduced.[139]

Some individuals suffering from PMS may have endometriosis or other conditions causing their symptoms; some may require pharmaceutical or surgical intervention. However, for the vast majority of women, conversion to a Wellness Forum-style diet, an appropriate exercise program, and other positive lifestyle changes will eliminate PMS naturally and quickly.

Pregnancy and Nutrition

Pregnancy often causes even women who are not particularly health-conscious to become interested in nutrition. The same diet The Wellness Forum recommends for everyone is also optimal for pregnancy, with the addition of slightly more calories.

We can all agree that nutrition during pregnancy is important, but one of the overlooked benefits of eating a proper diet during pregnancy is that a child's taste for food begins in the womb. The mother's diet during pregnancy and breastfeeding influences the baby's taste for foods when solids are introduced, according to a study reported in *Pediatrics*.[140]

What a great opportunity this presents for moms-to-be; eat lots of fruits, vegetables, and plant foods while you're pregnant and nursing, and it will be easier to get your child to do so when it is time to eat solid food. Another benefit is that moms can be in great shape and prepared for the demands of motherhood too!

Isolated Nutrients and Pregnancy

The best way for pregnant women to make sure they are getting the right nutrients every day is to eat a whole foods plant-based diet. With few exceptions, vitamins and other supplements are not beneficial.

Take folic acid, for example. It is true that folic acid has been shown to reduce neural tube defects, which result in deformities of the spinal cord, by half. But the benefit concerning risk reduction is expressed in relative rather than absolute terms, which is quite misleading. The risk of neural tube defects for women who do not take folic acid supplements is 2 in 1000. For women who do take them, the risk is about 1 in 2000. This is, indeed a 50% reduction in relative terms, but only a 1% reduction in absolute terms. So a woman who takes folic acid during pregnancy reduces the risk of neural tube defects by 1%. On the other hand, there are risks associated with taking folic acid supplements, including an increased risk of cancer.[141]

There really is no need for women who eat a well-structured plant-based diet to take folic acid supplements anyway. Folic acid comes from folate, which is found naturally in plants. Pregnant women get plenty of folate through diet and do not need to take it in supplement form.

Concerns about supplementation during pregnancy are not limited to folic acid. In a study that looked at the effects of Vitamins C and E on pre-eclampsia in high-risk women, the vitamins had no effect, and the women taking them had lower birth weight babies.[142]

To be fair, most doctors are prescribing prenatal vitamins and other supplements to pregnant women because they know most people do not eat an optimal diet, and it's the best option based on their training. However, the uncertainty about both the safety and efficacy of supplements makes eating a whole foods, plant-based diet the better choice.

Episiotomy - Another Useless Medical Procedure

According to research published in the *Journal of the American Medical Association,* episiotomy, an incision used in childbirth that is supposed to make delivery less stressful and reduce complications, actually has no benefits and increases complications.[143]

The study, which was the most comprehensive analysis of episiotomy ever done, concluded that the procedure increases the risk of tissue tears during delivery, leading to more pain, more stitches, and a longer recovery after childbirth. And, it increases the risk of sexual difficulties later.

More than 1 million women have this procedure annually. Although it can be helpful for speeding delivery when the baby's health is at risk, lead researcher Katherine Hartmann stated, "The evidence is clear: routine use of episiotomy is not supported by research and should stop."

Menopause

While many women dread menopause, it is actually sociologically beneficial. Traditionally, women have been the primary caregivers of children. Eliminating the potential for child bearing at 45 or 50 is nature's way of insuring that most women will live long enough to rear their own children.

The U.S. is one of the few cultures in the world in which menopause is considered to be a "disease" that requires medical attention and pharmaceutical intervention. In many other cultures, women do not experience symptoms at all during or after menopause.

American women not only experience more symptoms, but they tend to experience them for longer periods of time than women in other cultures.

In order to understand menopause and why some women experience symptoms, it's best to start with a discussion of the menstrual cycle. During the first half of the cycle, the hypothalamus secretes a messenger hormone to the pituitary gland, which signals the release of follicle stimulating hormone (FSH) and luteinizing hormone (LH). FSH stimulates the ovaries to develop and enlarge several follicles, and LH causes the uterine lining to thicken. The first part of the cycle is dominated by estrogen.

The second half of the cycle starts with ovulation. Progesterone is produced. In the absence of ovulation, no progesterone is produced. If the egg is not fertilized, the uterine lining is shed, resulting in a menstrual period.

The propensity to have difficulty during menopause actually begins during a woman's reproductive years. Most women experience abnormally high levels of estrogen as a result of poor diet, being overweight, and lack of physical activity. Although estrogen performs nearly 300 functions that are necessary for health, high estrogen levels can cause a number of health problems including impaired thyroid function, PMS, heavy menstrual bleeding, and increased risk of many types of cancer.

There are two ways in which women can experience menopause. One is a function of aging and the other is artificially induced from hysterectomy, chemotherapy for cancer treatment, or as a result of taking various prescription drugs.

When natural menopause begins, the number of eggs in the ovaries has decreased from 1-2 million to a few thousand. The menstrual cycle begins to vary and shorten. FSH levels increase. Ovarian production of hormones like estradiol and progesterone decreases. Eventually menstruation ceases.

This transition should occur without much fanfare, but it is common today for American women to experience symptoms like hot flashes, vaginal dryness, loss of libido, depression, weight gain and sleep disorders. These are symptoms of ill health, for which doctors often prescribe hormone replacement therapy (HRT).

But this is unnecessary – the human body was designed to produce all of the hormones needed for function for an entire lifetime. But diet and lifestyle habits, which lead to weight gain and other health issues, often compromise or alter hormone production. Taking HRT will suppress the symptoms but not address the cause of the disorder.

How Did We Get So Focused on HRT?

In 1943, Willard Allen extracted the first estrogenic product from horse urine. This was the basis for the blockbuster drug, Premarin which was marketed to relieve menopausal symptoms such as hot flashes.

Premarin sales soared when Dr. Robert Wilson popularized the idea that menopause was a condition for which women should be treated medically. In his book, *Feminine Forever*, Wilson

166

claimed to have placed thousands of women on estrogen replacement therapy. He stated that in order for women to remain attractive and vibrant, they *needed* estrogen replacement. In his book, he wrote:

> "The unthinkable truth must be faced that all postmenopausal women are castrates...From a practical point of view, a man remains a man until the very end. The situation with a woman is very different. Her ovaries become inadequate relatively early in life. She is the only mammal who cannot reproduce after middle age."

Although it is hard to believe, the book sold 100,000 copies and helped to make Premarin a best-selling drug. Millions of women were taught to think that HRT was needed in order to maintain health, and to restore youth and beauty after menopause. And Premarin resolved the symptoms of their poor diet and lifestyle choices, such as hot flashes.

Demand for HRT increased for a number of years until several studies showed increased risks of cancer and heart disease from taking the drugs. This eventually caused many women to seek other options, including bio-identical hormones.

The term "bio-identical hormones" refers to hormones that are usually derived from plant sources and are molecularly similar to human hormones. Most practitioners who prescribe bio-identical hormones use saliva or blood tests, and then hormones are custom compounded by a pharmacist. These hormones include estrone, estradiol, testosterone, and progesterone.

Women generally seek treatment with bio-identical hormone products to relieve symptoms of menopause, and because they believe that these products are safer.

But I have found no clear evidence that testing is effective for determining hormone levels and subsequently prescription s for hormone replacement. Saliva testing is not accurate, since very small levels of estrogen or progesterone are found in the saliva. It is almost a certainty that saliva testing will lead to a recommendation to supplement with hormones – great for compounding pharmacists, not so great for women.

Blood tests may be more accurate, but the problem with them is that hormone levels fluctuate from day to day and even from hour to hour, particularly in peri-menopausal women. This makes the results of these tests virtually meaningless.

Another issue is that I have been unable to locate any reliable information indicating how much supplemental hormone is needed in order to raise hormone levels. This makes prescribing hormone replacement a guessing game, and is often accompanied by trial and error.

Women in their 40's and 50's are often tested and told that their levels of estrogen and progesterone are low. This is normal; these lower levels accompany menopause. I have seen many reference charts in which the goal seems to "treat" women in order to restore their hormone levels to those of women much younger. This is not a good idea; we know that there are serious risks in using pharmaceutical HRT to accomplish this objective and we don't have safety data on bio-identical hormones.

Last but not least, bio-identical hormone replacement does not address the underlying cause of menopausal symptoms; it just relieves symptoms.

Is Hormone Replacement Ever a Viable Alternative?

The severity of symptoms may sometimes necessitate hormone replacement therapy, but it is best to make this a short-term strategy. Health problems are best resolved by looking for underlying causes and resolving them, rather than suppressing symptoms. Your body was designed to produce all of the hormones you need for your entire life, and if production is impaired, restoring its ability to do so should be the goal of treatment. Additionally, long-term use of hormone replacement therapy, synthetic or natural, can gradually reduce or eliminate a woman's natural production of hormones.

What About Progesterone Creams?

It is natural for your body to produce less progesterone as you age. When your body stops preparing for pregnancy every month, the need for progesterone decreases. The reason why progesterone creams "work" is they help to counteract abnormally high estrogen levels. The better solution, however, is to address the underlying reasons for these high estrogen levels and lower them.

However, many medical professionals have attributed the symptoms of peri-menopause and menopause to a progesterone deficiency, which they contend can be remedied by using progesterone creams.

There are numerous over-the-counter creams available today. They can be purchased in drug stores, health food stores, through direct sales agents, and through the internet. Many of these products contain toxic chemicals. This is particularly dangerous when you are applying a substance to your skin, as anything applied to the skin is absorbed directly into the bloodstream and bypasses the liver's detoxification system. This means you are getting a much more potent effect from the chemicals than if you were to ingest them orally.

The active compound in progesterone in its natural state is too large to be absorbed through the skin. "Natural" progesterone creams made from plant sources have been chemically altered in order to allow them to be absorbed,
which means they are no longer "natural."

I advise against the use of these products too.

Managing Menopause Naturally

The best way to manage menopause is through a combination of proper diet, exercise, stress reduction, adequate relaxation, sleep, and nurturing relationships.

Generally, women who follow a diet close to the one recommended by The Wellness Forum consistently for a number of years, maintain normal weight, get regular exercise, and learn to control stress, can expect to have a relatively uneventful menopause. Women who begin making healthy lifestyle and dietary changes during menopause may experience symptoms for a period of time until their body chemistry changes from improved nutrition and exercise.

Food choices can assist in properly regulating hormone production. For example, vegetarians have lower levels of estradiol and estrone, which results in fewer menopausal symptoms and a lower risk of cancer. Diets high in animal protein and fat, on the other hand, raise hormone levels and cause more severe menopausal symptoms.

A byproduct of our modern lifestyles is that we are more sedentary than any population that has ever lived on earth. This has terrible implications for overall health, but also aggravates symptoms of menopause. Weight gain is often related to inactivity, and becomes worse during menopause. Increasing physical activity is one way to improve body composition and appearance.

A well-structured exercise program can reduce the amount or severity of hot flashes and night sweats, and result in restful sleep.

Exercise has been proven to be as effective as drug treatment for mild to moderate depression, another common symptoms associated with menopause. And, exercise lowers estrogen levels, reducing the risk of many forms of cancer.

An appropriate exercise plan means spending 45-60 minutes 5-6 days per week engaged in physical activity in your target heart zone. Two sessions per week should be allocated to strength training, 3-4 to some form of aerobic exercise, and if you like yoga, it is a wonderful way to stretch muscles and gain flexibility.

Stress exacerbates symptoms of menopause and contributes to health problems overall. Stress is also one of the causes of adrenal insufficiency, which can exacerbate menopausal symptoms. A combination of eating well and exercise can contribute greatly to reducing stress.

But sometimes life circumstances are difficult and therapy may be needed. If this is the case, I recommend finding a good Cognitive Behavioral Therapist. CBT is a very effective form of therapy that works within a few sessions, and has a very low recidivism rate. Good CBT practitioners are very conservative about the use of drugs.

Menopausal Weight Gain

Weight gain is prevalent in middle-aged women. Although this is often assumed to be a result of hormone fluctuations, it is more likely the cumulative effects of years of poor diet and lack of enough physical activity.

Dr. Neal Barnard and his colleagues showed that a low-fat vegan diet resulted in significant weight loss in women between the ages of 44 and 73, the ages at which women are often told their hormones are responsible for their weight gain.[144] The participants were randomly assigned to either a low-fat vegan diet, or a more traditional low-fat diet. They were specifically asked not to alter their exercise patterns during the duration of the study. The women on the low-fat vegan diet lost an average of 13 pounds in 14 weeks.

With few exceptions, weight gain can be avoided, or excess weight can be lost with the right diet and exercise habits.

Withdrawing from HRT

You may have decided after reading this material that you want to discontinue using hormone replacement.
If you were told to take HRT without ever experiencing symptoms, you may not have any problems withdrawing. If HRT was prescribed to address symptoms, they may reappear for a time after you discontinue the use of the drugs.

If you are overweight, have not been engaged in an appropriate amount of physical activity, or have not been practicing dietary excellence™, you are more likely to experience unpleasant symptoms after discontinuing HRT. These symptoms eventually resolve with the right diet and lifestyle choices.

Osteoporosis – The Real Story

Every year, millions of women have a DXA scan and are told that they have osteopenia or osteoporosis. But these diagnoses are incorrect most of the time.

Before the 1990's, testing for osteoporosis was only recommended when a patient presented with fragile bones or unexplainable fractures or breaks. Bone scans were expensive and were therefore not routinely performed. The diagnosis of osteoporosis at that time meant weakened bones that were more inclined to fracture.

This presented a problem for the drug companies, which had developed drugs to treat osteoporosis. Based on the criteria at that time, the drugs were rarely prescribed, making the market for them very small. In response, the always-enterprising drug companies decided to change both the method of diagnosis and the diagnostic criteria. A marketing guru hired by Merck, the maker of Fosomax, was the chief architect of the plan.

In 1992, the World Health Organization organized a meeting of experts on bone health for the purpose of redefining diagnostic and treatment parameters for osteoporosis. This meeting was funded by the drug companies, an automatic red flag in my opinion.[145]

The experts at this meeting were well aware that some thinning of the bones and the loss of bone mineral density is normal for women as they age. More dense bones are needed to support pregnancy during a woman's reproductive years; after a woman's child-bearing years, bone mineral density declines. In spite of this knowledge, the experts re-defined osteoporosis as a loss of bone mineral density. According to those in attendance, an arbitrary level of BMD loss had to be chosen, since there was no evidence that this loss was really anything other than a normal function of aging. But the net effect of this meeting was that a normal marker of aging was used as the definition of the disease, which guaranteed millions of potential customers for drugs that previously were appropriate for only a few.

The panel also determined that those patients who were "borderline" and did not qualify for a diagnosis of osteoporosis would be labeled as having a new condition called osteopenia, or "pre-osteoporosis."[146]

In order to capitalize on this great opportunity, Merck's marketing department directed the development of cheap bone scanning devices that could be easily placed in doctors' offices, developed leasing programs that made it easier for doctors to have the machines, and even helped to pass a law mandating that Medicare reimburse for the bone scans. In addition to full-dose Fosomax to treat the now mythical diagnosis of osteoporosis, Merck developed a lower dose to treat the new mythical condition called osteopenia.

Loss of bone mineral density is not only a normal biomarker of aging, but is also a poor predictor of fracture risk. Several studies have examined this relationship and reached this conclusion; one that looked at several populations and over 2000 fractures concluded, "We do not recommend a program of screening menopausal women for osteoporosis by measuring bone density."[147]

Yet most women are advised to start having bone scans in their 40's; most will eventually be told that they have osteopenia or osteoporosis; and most of those women are told that they need to take drugs to treat their "condition."

Does Anyone *Really* Have Osteoporosis?

This information does not mean that no one develops osteoporosis. Some people do have it. The disease, when it does occur, results from a condition in the body called metabolic acidosis, a byproduct of eating the Standard American Diet, with lots of meat, dairy, and processed and refined foods. In an attempt to neutralize the acidity, the body releases calcium, a buffer, from the bones.

Osteoporosis can also result from taking pharmaceutical drugs like steroids, and from malabsorption, which is common in people who have celiac disease and other gastrointestinal disorders.

173

Then What Causes Fractures?

Falling presents the biggest risk of fracture, not bone mineral density, and the type and trajectory of many falls experienced by the elderly would cause fractures even in very young people.

At least half of the hip fractures in women over the age of 80 are not a result of reduced bone mineral density. They are a result of the way people fall, the position of the hip at the time of the fall (standing vs. squatting at the time of the fall, for example), and the structure of the hip. Asian women have shorter hip axes than white women; therefore they will suffer fewer hip fractures regardless of bone mineral density.

Additionally, low body weight, epilepsy, poor circulation, taking prescription drugs, poor coordination, poor eyesight, lack of balance, and dementia are responsible for many falls. In other words, an increased propensity to fall causes fractures, and this increased risk is largely due to declining health and taking prescription drugs as people age.

Treating the Mythical Disease

Once diagnosed, women are told that they must be treated in order to avoid becoming bedridden as a result of fractures and broken bones. Bisphosphonate drugs are usually recommended. These include Fosomax, Actonel and Boniva. These drugs are notoriously ineffective and increasing evidence is showing that they are harmful.

Fosomax is reported to reduce fracture rates by 44%, which sounds impressive. However, this is only because Merck, like most drug companies, reports the benefits of its drugs in relative, rather than absolute terms.

The Fracture Intervention Trial showed that after 3 years, 2.1% of women who took Fosomax had fractures, as compared to 3.8% of women who took a placebo. This is, indeed, a 44% reduction in relative terms. But in absolute terms, this is a 1.7% reduction in risk for the person taking the drug, not a 44% reduction in risk; a very small benefit.[148] The same statistical sleight of hand is used to report the benefits of other drugs in the same class.

Fosomax works by blocking the effects of osteoclast cells, which slows bone resorption. This is why some women who take Fosomax show increases in bone density during the first year or so that they take the drug.

However, this is a problem since osteoclasts remove older, weakened bone, which is then replaced with new bone through the action of osteoblasts. Osteoblasts respond to the activity of osteoclasts. Interfering with this process actually causes bone fragility and can increase the likelihood of fractures. To date, there have been no long-term studies examining the effects of taking the drug for an extended period of time on bone health.

Fosomax deposits in the bone and remains there for more than 10 years, so discontinuing the use of the drug does not immediately stop its action.

There are serious side effects from taking Fosomax, with 1 in 3 women reporting severe digestive problems that include irritation, inflammation, or ulceration of the esophagus. Women have to stick with a strict regimen for taking the drug to avoid some side effects. The drug must be taken on an empty stomach and women cannot eat for two hours after taking it. It is necessary to sit upright for 30 minutes because of the risk of irritating, or even burning holes in the esophagus if even a tiny amount of the drug enters the esophageal tube. 56% of women fail to comply with the instructions.

Actonel works in much the same way as Fosomax. In addition to studies showing that there is also minimal benefit from taking this drug, there are serious side effects too. Potential damage to the esophagus, back pain, nausea, headache, edema, diarrhea, and abdominal pain are common.

The drug manufacturers have responded to increasing reports of serious side effects by developing versions of their products that can be taken monthly or even annually instead of daily.

Even more concerning, however, is the increasing evidence that these drugs increase the risk of fractures, the very problem they are supposed to prevent.

According to a study published in the *Journal of Bone and Mineral Research*[149] in April 2000, taking Fosomax significantly suppressed bone remodeling and increased microdamage accumulation. Bone toughness declined by 20% in the group treated with the drug.

In June 2008, Dr. Dean Lorich, associate director of orthopedic trauma surgery at New York Presbyterian/Weill Cornell and the Hospital for Special Surgery published a study in the *Journal of Orthopedic Trauma*[150] reporting 20 cases in which a fracture sheared the thighbone with little or no trauma. 19 of those patients had been taking Fosomax for an average of 6.9 years. This is noteworthy because the femur bone is the strongest bone in the body. A fracture of this bone without impact is almost unheard of. Lorich told the *New York Times* that doctors should monitor long-term users of the drug, consider advising patients to take time off from it, and when fractures do occur, that surgeons should be alerted that the patients may require more aggressive treatment since the bones may be slower to heal.

Osteonecrosis of the jaw (ONJ) is a painful condition in which portions of the jaw bone die, the gums become infected, and fragments of the dead and decaying bone are exposed. As the condition progresses, eating can be very difficult and the decaying bone can cause a horrible odor. The condition is not easily treated – in addition to surgery to remove the dead bone, the mouth can take up to two years to completely heal.

Formerly considered a very rare condition, dentists started reporting an increasing number of cases of ONJ in 2003. These early cases were cancer patients who took bisphosphonate drugs in an effort to keep their cancers from metastasizing to the bones.

However, more and more non-cancer patients taking these drugs are developing osteonecrosis of the jaw. The companies making the drugs continue to insist that the incidence is rare, but in response to the increasing number of cases being reported, a study was conducted and published in the *Journal of the American Dental Association*.[151]

The researchers looked at the dental records of 13,000 patients at the University of Southern California's dental school clinic. They identified 208 patients taking Fosomax and of them 4% had ONJ.

According to lead researcher Parish Sedghizadeh, "As we get more patients with 10 or 15 years experience with bisphosphonates, we'll likely see more cases. We really haven't hit the top of the curve."

These drugs are dangerous and ineffective, and most often used to treat made-up diseases marketed to the public by the drug companies. A better alternative is to improve diet and lifestyle habits in order to preserve bone health. Your bones were designed to last as long as you do if you take care of them properly!

Men's Health: Proper Feeding and Care of the Prostate

The Prostate

The prostate consists of several glands encased in an outer shell. It is the size of a walnut and surrounds the beginning of the urethra. The prostate produces some, but not all of the semen, and the fluid that accompanies semen, and stimulates the activity of sperm, facilitating reproduction.

The incidence of both prostate diseases and cancer have increased in the U.S., another byproduct of the Standard American Diet. if you are diagnosed with prostate cancer, your urologist will almost certainly recommend that you receive treatment. By the age of 80, 25% of all American men have undergone some form of treatment for prostate cancer. About 500,000 surgeries are performed each year, most of them with life-altering and negative consequences, such as impotence and incontinence.

Prostate Disease

Prostate infections are caused by microorganisms that penetrate the outer shell of the prostate. Straining due to constipation is one way for bacteria to enter the prostate through the lymph system. External irritations such as catheters, sex, anal sex, sex with women who have yeast infections, venereal disease, and flukes (parasitic worms usually picked up in foreign countries) are some of the other ways that a prostate infection can develop.

Symptoms of infection include fever, chills, penile discharges, and severe pain. Treatment includes sulfa drugs such as Bactrim and Septra. Occasionally, surgery may be required if prostate stones develop.

Prostate congestion results when excess fluid, which is normally released during sex, builds up inside the prostate gland. Causes can include intense sex, or extended periods of abstinence. Prostate massage and/or sex are the best options for resolving congestion.

Benign prostate enlargement is referred to as BPH (Benign Prostate Hyperplasia or Hypertrophy). The first symptoms are usually trouble urinating or urinating frequently because the enlarged gland places pressure on the urethra and the neck of the bladder. The condition is only fatal if it results in a urinary tract blockage.

Untreated BPH can result in recurring bladder infections, diverticula in the bladder, high blood pressure, blood in the urine and painful ejaculation.

Treatment for BPH includes watchful waiting (it will sometimes resolve with diet and lifestyle changes), balloon dilation and urethral prostheses, drug treatment to control testosterone production, radiation, surgery, and castration. The side effects of drug treatment include hot flashes, loss of libido, impotence, and gastrointestinal problems. The side effects of radiation are also significant and include destruction of healthy prostate tissue.

Following any type of invasive procedure to the prostate, between 50% and 100% of men will experience impotence or have difficulty having an erection, depending on age. 25% will end up permanently incontinent.

What Causes Prostate Disease?

Diet and lifestyle choices affect the production of testosterone, which affects prostate health. The condition of the cardiovascular system influences blood flow, which affects the prostate too.

A study conducted at George Mason University showed that a Westernized diet increases the risk of prostate cancer.[152] The researchers reported that the highest rates of prostate cancer are in Sweden and the U.S., while the lowest rates are in China and India.

They concluded, "In large population studies performed in over 60 countries, as well as in prospective cohort studies, intake of dairy products, red meat, and total dietary fat have been found to be positively correlated with increased risk of prostate cancer. In contrast, consumption of soy products, fiber-containing foods, cruciferous vegetables and lycopene, have been reported to be inversely associated with prostate cancer risk. These studies suggest that predominantly plant-based diets that are high in fiber and phytonutrients and low in fat and saturated fat, favorably influence health outcomes for prostate cancer patients."

A study published in the *British Journal of Nutrition* concluded that high fat intake of any kind may be a risk factor for the development of prostate cancer.[153] The study included 512 men with prostate cancer and 838 healthy controls. Those consuming the highest levels of fat in the diet had a 153% increased incidence of prostate cancer when compared to men eating the least fat. The risks were the same for saturated, monounsaturated, and polyunsaturated fat.

Regular consumption of dairy products can double the risk of prostate cancer. Growth hormones used in dairy production, including rBGH, increase milk output in cows. But rBGH also increases Insulin-Like Growth Factor (IGF-1) levels in humans, which in turn increases prostate cancer risk.

The Health Professionals Follow-up Study[154] included 47, 781 health care professionals and concluded that men who consumed more than two servings per day of cow's milk products increased their risk of cancer by 60% as compared to men who consumed no cow's milk. More than 80% of the milk consumed by study participants was low-fat or no-fat milk, adding to the body of evidence that suggests that dairy protein, rather than fat, is the major culprit in the development of disease.

Another study concluded that higher calcium intake resulted not only in increased risk of cancer, but also higher risk of advanced and fatal cancers.[155] Men who consumed over 2000 mg of calcium per day had more than two times the risk of advanced or fatal prostate cancer as compared to men who consumed less than 750 mg per day.

The Physicians Health Study concluded that men who consumed 2.5 servings of dairy products per day had a significantly increased risk of prostate cancer as compared to those who consumed less than .5 serving daily.[156]

Obesity is another factor for prostate cancer risk. Of course, obese men often consume lots of animal protein and saturated

183

fat, which are known risk factors. And adipose tissue contributes to higher levels of sex hormones, including testosterone. Maintaining a lean body seems to offer some protection – men with less aggressive tumors tend to be leaner than those with more aggressive forms of prostate cancer.

Many supplements commonly used by men can increase the risk of prostate cancer, and supplements that were thought to have a protective effect have not proven to be effective. These include:

- DHEA, often marketed as an anti-aging aid, increases testosterone production.
- Anabolic steroids, which are used by athletes to increase muscle mass, can stimulate abnormal growth of prostate cells.
- Testosterone is often taken by men to increase libido and improve muscle mass, and can increase the risk of prostate cancer.
- The SELECT trial involved 35,000 men age 50 and older who took Vitamin E, selenium, a combination of both, or placebo. The study, which looked at the potential for supplements to reduce the risk of prostate cancer, was supposed to run through 2011, with patients being followed for an average of 7 years. It was stopped early because the men taking only Vitamin E experienced a slightly higher risk of developing prostate cancer; and those men taking only selenium experienced a slightly higher rate of diabetes.[157]
- A large study involving 14,641 participants showed that taking vitamins C and E did not reduce the risk of prostate cancer.[158]
- Multivitamins, thought by many people to provide an "insurance policy" against a less than optimal diet, may increase the risk of developing prostate cancer.[159]

PSA Testing

Prostate cancer is almost always primary – it starts in the prostate gland rather than metastasizing there from another part of the body. Every year, 200,000 American men are diagnosed with it, and 30,000 men die of it.

Prostate cancer is usually diagnosed following a blood test showing elevated PSA levels. Prostate Specific Antigen is a protein produced by the prostate. It is believed to break down coagulated semen, and may provide some protection against cancer.

Both normal and cancerous cells produce PSA, but cancer cells produce larger amounts of it, which is why an elevated PSA count may indicate cancer.

But PSA tests are unreliable. By the time a man is 60, the incidence of cancer is the same with or without elevated PSA, according to a study published in *Urology*.[160]

Studies show that populations that get prostate cancer screening regularly show no reduction in prostate cancer deaths as compared to those that do not.[161]

Here is how PSA scores are generally interpreted:
- Less than 1 - 1% chance of cancer progressing in 3 years.
- Between 1-2 – 4% chance of PSA increasing to 4 or higher within 4 years
- Between 2-4 – considered normal but should be watched.
- Between 4-10 – 25-30% chance of having prostate cancer.
- 10 or higher – 70-80% chance of having prostate cancer.

It is common for doctors to recommend a biopsy in response to high PSA levels, which is usually painful and can result in infection. And many of these biopsies are not necessary.

Researchers at Memorial Sloan Kettering in New York City determined that elevated PSA tests should always be confirmed with follow-up testing prior to doing anything else,[162] since these follow-up tests often show reduced or even normal PSA levels.

According to Dr. Michael Barry of Massachusetts General Hospital, "The bottom line is we still don't know whether PSA (testing) does more good than harm." An honest statement, but millions of healthy men will still be advised to have a PSA test this year, in spite of risks that include false positives, unnecessary biopsies, and the anxiety that accompanies a possible diagnosis of cancer.

Many early detection tests, not just PSA testing, are being called into question. By the time many cancers are detectable, they have been developing for a long time. The more tests administered, the greater the chance of a false positive, while negative results give people a false sense of security that they are really ok and can continue with their current habits.

Most of the time, early diagnoses are followed by ridiculously over-zealous treatment, with watchful waiting rarely part of the plan. Additionally, traditional treatment for metastasized cancer is notoriously ineffective, subjecting patients to expensive and usually awful drug therapies and procedures which rarely extend life and usually compromise quality of remaining life.

There is not one randomized trial that shows a survival advantage that justifies removal of the prostate or most other aggressive treatments such as radiation therapy and radioactive seed implantation. In low-risk patients, aggressive treatment is not necessary, and in high-risk cases, the treatment does not save lives.

The only strategy that works to save preserve your prostate and protect your health is dietary excellence™ and optimal habits. It is always easier to prevent than to treat cancer of any type.

What to do if You Have Prostate Disease

Sometimes the best approach is watchful waiting. A study followed 14,516 men diagnosed between 1992 and 2002 who agreed to watchful waiting instead of treatment. The results showed a 10-year overall survival of 94%.[163]

If you've been diagnosed, start practicing dietary excellence and optimal lifestyle habits now. There are good reasons to consider drugs and surgery as last resorts, rather than the first line of treatment, and to focus on dietary improvement first.

The September 2005 issue of *Urology* featured the results of a randomized, controlled trial that demonstrated the impact of diet and lifestyle changes on the progression of prostate cancer.

A research team led by Dr. Peter Carroll, Chair of the department of urology at the University of California and Dr. Dean Ornish, Founder and President of the Preventive Medicine Research Institute in San Francisco selected 93 men with biopsy-proven prostate cancer who had decided not to have conventional treatment.

The men were divided into two groups, with one group placed on a vegan diet consisting of fruit, vegetables, whole grains, soy, and legumes. Additionally, the men took vitamins and mineral supplements, participated in moderate aerobic exercise, yoga and meditation, and attended a weekly support group session. These men did not receive any conventional treatments such as surgery, radiation, or chemotherapy during the study period.

The control group continued their current lifestyle habits. Six of them eventually decided to pursue conventional treatment after their disease progressed.

After one year, PSA levels decreased in the vegan group, while those in the control group experienced an increase. There were correlations noted between degree of dietary change and positive changes in PSA.

Additionally, the researchers found that serum from the vegan participants inhibited prostate tumor growth in vitro by 70%, while serum from the control group inhibited prostate tumor growth by only 9%.

Dr. Ornish commented. "Changes in diet and lifestyle that we found in earlier research could reverse the progression of coronary heart disease may also affect the progression of prostate cancer as well."

Dr. Ornish is referring to his extensive studies involving the use of a similar diet and lifestyle that was proven to reverse heart disease. 90% of his cardiovascular patients were able to avoid bypass surgery and drug therapies at the end of one year, and compliance on his diet was actually better than for patients following the more moderate recommendations of the American Heart Association.

Researchers are continuing to monitor these prostate patients to determine the effects of dietary changes on morbidity and mortality.[164]

By contrast, the results from conventional treatment leave a lot to be desired.

Androgen deprivation therapy involves reducing male hormone levels through either castration or drug treatment. It is now widely used to treat many types of prostate cancer.

A study published in the *Journal of the American Medical Association*[165] showed that patients treated with androgen therapy experienced lower prostate cancer-specific survival and no increase in 10-year overall survival. This is significant in view of the side effects associated with androgen deprivation therapy, which can include impotence, incontinence, increased risk of fractures, and other degenerative conditions. And, androgen deprivation therapy is expensive – the expense to Medicare alone for this treatment is $1.2 billion per year.

A study published in the *New England Journal of Medicine* examined the efficacy of radical prostatectomy vs. watchful waiting in early prostate cancer.[166] After 10 years of follow-up the researchers concluded that surgery reduced the risk of death by only 5%.

Prostate cancer treatments almost always have negative side effects. One study looked at outcomes in men, half of whom had their prostates surgically removed; the others were treated with external beam radiation, external beam radiation with androgen suppression therapy, brachytherapy, or brachytherapy combined with either external beam radiation or androgen suppression.[167]

50% of the surgery group, 31% in the radiation group and 30% in the brachytherapy group reported sexual function to be a moderate or big problem. 12% of the surgery group, 14% of the radiotherapy group and 18% of the brachytherapy group complained of urinary irritation or obstruction. 11% of the patients receiving radiotherapy and 10% of those receiving brachytherapy complained of bowel or rectal dysfunction. Obese men were more likely to suffer adverse side effects than normal weight men.

The fact is that 10 years after diagnosis, 85% of men with prostate cancer will not have died from it. When you take into consideration the dreadful outcomes of most of the common drugs and procedures, including impotence and incontinence, there is no real reason for most men to have them. Dietary excellence can often slow the growth of this already slow-growing cancer so that most men will die *with* prostate cancer rather than of it. This is certainly the case with Asian men, almost all of whom have prostate cancer at death but few of whom ever receive treatment for it.

Should I Have a Vasectomy?

Vasectomy blocks the vas deferens and keeps sperm out of the seminal fluid. Whether or not the procedure is advisable is a source of disagreement among medical professionals.

A study of 3000 men in Scotland who had a vasectomy showed an increase in testicular cancer risk.[168]

According to the textbook Campbell's Urology, "The brunt of pressure induced damage after a vasectomy falls on the epididymis and efferent tubules...It is likely that, in time, all vasectomized men develop 'blowouts' in either the epididymis or efferent ducts."[169]

When rupturing does occur, sperm enter the bloodstream, and antibodies are created. Continuous stimulation of the immune system in this manner can lead to autoimmune diseases. One byproduct of autoimmune disease can be the formation of cysts in the scrotum. These cysts sometimes need to be removed surgically.

Vasectomy is generally elected as a form of birth control. Although it is promoted as a low-risk procedure, the adverse consequences should be considered, as well as other and perhaps better alternatives.

Diet-Centered Health Care

a model for the future

Conditions Positively Affected by Diet-Centered Health Care

Which medical conditions can be expected to respond positively to plant-based nutrition? According to Dr. John McDougall, all of them will. He says, "People always get better. If they're eating the rich Western diet and you put them on the right food, they always get better... How many cigarette smokers do you know that quit smoking and didn't get better? How many hard-core alcoholics do you know that quit alcohol and didn't get better? The same thing with the food. You take people that are being fueled improperly, they're living on meat and dairy, and you correct that, and what happens is they get better. They essentially *all* get better."

One of the best things about getting better with diet and lifestyle is that this places the patient in control of his or her health; with this model of health care, doctors and patients are partners in the process, working together toward health improvement.

Scientific Evidence for the Use of a Plant-Based Diet in Treating Disease

The discussion of appropriate treatments for degenerative conditions should always be based on scientific evidence. One of my major criticisms of traditional treatments is that published research shows that most of them are ineffective and many of them are harmful.

The scientific literature includes excellent data on the effects of diet on diabetes and coronary artery disease. Dr. Caldwell Esselstyn followed his original group of cardiovascular patients for over 12 years, making his study the longest ever conducted on the effects of diet on coronary artery disease. There is a small but growing body of evidence about the effects of diet on cancer. And there is evidence that diet can stop the progression of multiple sclerosis. Dr. Roy Swank followed his multiple sclerosis patients after placing them on a low-fat diet for 34 years, and published amazing results from dietary intervention.

Unfortunately, I cannot cite similar studies of this length and quality for conditions like infertility, gastrointestinal disorders and asthma. Yet I think it would be a mistake to totally discount the growing number of stories from people documenting essentially the same experiences using diet to recover from many different diseases, particularly since these stories are consistent with a large number of peer-reviewed, published articles on diet and health. It is my hope that the information in this section will lead to further discussion and interest in conducting long-term studies on the effect of plant-based nutrition on many degenerative conditions.

If I wait until these studies are finished and published to talk about the positive effects of plant-based nutrition, this book would be published in 2030 instead of 2010. I think it's time to start talking about these issues now because there are many who will be helped by this information, and because there is no evidence that adopting a low-fat, well-structured plant-based diet has any detrimental effects.

The information in this book should not be taken as personal medical advice; decisions about your health and how to treat degenerative conditions should be made with a qualified health care practitioner who is familiar with your health history. If you are taking medications for conditions like diabetes or hypertension, you should consult with a physician prior to changing your diet, as your medications may need to be reduced and sometimes even eliminated, and you should be medically supervised while doing so.

On the following pages you will read about some of the more common conditions plaguing Americans today. Most likely you or someone you know is struggling with one or more of these issues. In addition to basic information about how the wrong diet causes these conditions and the right diet can help, you'll read stories of real people who have succeeded in re-gaining their health with plant-based nutrition.

Weight Gain: A Growing Problem

Close to 60% of the population is overweight or obese, with more people being categorized as obese each year. In fact, today overweight Americans outnumber those who are normal weight.[170]

The obesity epidemic not only affects adults, but it is affecting children now too. According to The National Center for Health Statistics, almost one third of Americans twenty years of age and older are obese; the same trend is occurring in children as young as three.[171] This is a tragic set of circumstances for children. Not only can these children expect to experience health issues related to their weight, but obese children rate their quality of life as slightly worse than children undergoing chemotherapy for cancer.[172]

Obesity has become an expensive problem. According to the U.S. Centers for Disease Control, we spend about $147 billion every year on obesity-related illnesses and complications because obese people are not only more likely to develop degenerative conditions, they are more likely to die of them too. What is causing this recent increase in the obesity rate?

Scientists have tried in vain to find "obesity genes" which would account for this rapid explosion in obesity rates. But as you've read earlier, it's not your genes that are responsible for your health; it's your diet.

On the surface, it would seem that maintaining the right weight is really quite simple. You can't eat more calories than you burn each day. To lose weight, you have to eat fewer calories than you burn daily. This "common knowledge" leads to the belief that limiting calories, or portion control, is all that is required in order to lose weight. That's the basis for most weight loss plans, but for most people, this strategy does not work.

Humans are designed, just like all creatures on the earth, to eat enough food to sustain their weight and daily activities, *provided we are eating the right foods for our species.* The problem is that in recent decades, we have had unprecedented access to foods that are not appropriate for us, and at incredibly and sometimes artificially low prices, making it very easy to eat too much of the wrong types of food. These foods are concentrated in fat, sugar, salt and most important, calories. Many of them contain little or no fiber, which makes them even easier to overeat.

Under normal circumstances, nature provides humans with a very efficient mechanism that tells us when it is time to eat (we feel hungry) and when to stop (we feel full). There are two mechanisms that notify us that we are full. Stretch receptors tell the brain that there is enough bulk in the stomach. Nutrient receptors detect the calorie density. Both mechanisms are important for survival.

For example, if you eat a pound of vegetables, your stomach is likely to be full, but you will still not be satisfied because the nutrient receptors detect that there is not enough calorie density to the food (a pound of vegetables has only 100 calories). On the other hand, eating a large salad with beans and rice provides about 400-500 calories, which not only fills the stomach but provides enough calorie density to satisfy the nutrient receptors, resulting in a feeling of satiety.

These mechanisms have helped humans to eat precisely the right amounts of food with the right calorie content, long before they had the ability to count calories or to measure the nutrient values of food.

The foods most Americans eat most of the time (animal foods, oils, fat, and processed foods) have little to no fiber and are very calorie-dense, which facilitates overeating from a calorie standpoint. It takes about one liter of food to fill the stomach and provide a feeling of satiety. Cheese has no fiber and is high in calories; it takes 3400 calories to fill the stomach with cheese. A liter of vegetables and beans is high in fiber and requires only 400 calories to fill the stomach. Obviously eating high-calorie, low-fiber foods like cheese until you feel full will lead to weight gain, and research confirms this. When people eating meals lower in calorie density, like beans and vegetables, were compared to people eating meals comprised of higher-calorie foods, those eating the higher-calorie foods consumed twice as many calories in order to satisfy their hunger.[173]

This is why portion control does not work; putting the food on a smaller plate, putting the fork down in between bites, and other "tricks" of the diet trade do not help people to experience satiety while eating small portions of calorie-dense foods.

When eating a well-structured plant-based diet, you can eat as much as you want, whenever you want, and you will not gain weight. There is no calorie counting, no weighing and measuring, no portion control, and no willpower involved. You will feel full and satisfied, and the fiber content of the food will prevent overeating. For example, a bowl of black bean soup and a large salad has about 14 grams of fiber. Try to eat four servings, and you'll explode.

If you are overweight and adopt this diet, you will lose about 2 pounds per week until you reach your ideal weight, and once there, you'll maintain it easily and naturally.

Barbara J. Mathison's Story

From the ages of two to twelve, I lived on dairy farms, with cows, pigs, chickens, and rabbits. Animal foods made up the largest part of my diet. For 56 years I was from 30 to 110 pounds overweight, and I frequently had both physical and mental problems. Throughout those years I did many weight loss programs including high-carb, high-protein, fruit-only diets, Atkins, Weight Watchers, TopFast, TOPS, various supplements, and even took weight loss drugs looking for the "silver bullet."

I was successful in losing weight from time to time; I was signed as Liza Minelli's official look-alike in 1986 after losing 70 pounds.

In October 1996 I discovered a walnut size lump in my left breast. By March 1, 1999 the tumor had grown to the size of a large avocado, and I could no longer ignore it. I was eventually referred to a breast cancer surgeon and was diagnosed with Stage III breast cancer. I had seven treatments with chemotherapy, followed by a mastectomy. During my treatments, I ate more fruit and vegetables, but went back to eating more meat and dairy during the next several years after my treatment.

My health continued to decline. I had a mini-stroke that resulted in retinal vein occlusion; I was taking medication for high blood pressure, high cholesterol and pain; I was diagnosed with fibromyalgia; I weighed 170 pounds and was continuing to gain more weight.

The last straw was that my mother was living with us, and taking 19 pills every day. One of her doctors told me that was what I had to look forward to. I said "NO."

On May 7, 2007 I became a vegan. I read *The China Study* and knew then that I would never eat animal products again. I also knew I didn't have to be like my mother.

Within 4 months after starting my new diet, I no longer had any pains in my body, I no longer needed my blood pressure meds, I *terminated* 40 pounds, and my cholesterol went down 103 points. I had no more constipation, which I had suffered from my entire life; and my lab work showed I was healthy! I know that I would not have had to go through all of the health, mental, and weight issues, and would not have lost my breast if I had adopted a plant-based lifestyle earlier.

I've stayed on this diet and I continue to get healthier - even my eyesight has almost returned to normal. My eye doctor has agreed it could be related to what I eat! In fact she and her husband have joined the Vegetarian Society of Utah of which I am president.

It is easy to maintain my 120-pound weight and my new size 4 shape, and I am never hungry or crave anything but delicious plant-based foods. I walk 30 minutes per day and do Tai Chi 3 days per week. I lead a very active life. My everyday life has changed completely. In addition to being President of the Vegetarian Society of Utah and publishing the organization's newsletter, I operate a Health and Motivational Speaker business. I work from 8:00AM to 10:00PM (at least) every day and love it.

I advise everyone to go to events featuring lectures by experts like Dr. Campbell, Dr. McDougall, Dr. Popper and others, to get their newsletters, and to read their books. Information and support are essential for success. Meeting most of the key "players" in whole food nutrition has also helped me feel confident and to keep me on the right path.

Heart Disease

Healthy arteries are strong and elastic and lined with endothelial tissue that is smooth like Teflon. The endothelial cells produce a substance called nitric oxide, a vasodilator. Nitric oxide keeps the arteries open, which allows the unrestricted flow of blood through the cardiovascular system.

When levels of fat in the blood begin to rise, the endothelial cells begin to change, eventually becoming "sticky." Fat and cholesterol begin to stick to the artery walls, and white blood cells attempt to "clean up" the increasing levels of fat and cholesterol by ingesting it. As more of them gather and become filled with fat, a plaque is formed. A fibrous "cap" develops over the plaque, which is covered by a single layer of endothelial cells. Damage to the endothelial cells results in reduced nitric oxide production, and the vessels begin to narrow. Additionally, the inside (lumen) of the arteries narrow as plaque forms and grows. High blood pressure is one byproduct of this arterial constriction.

The serious problems begin when the white blood cells, which are filled with LDL cholesterol, begin to secrete chemicals that can gradually erode the thin cap of the plaques. The force of blood running over these thinned caps can cause them to rupture. The pus from the plaques then oozes into the bloodstream, activating platelets that try to contain the damage by clotting. Within a very short period of time, the entire artery can become blocked. The blockage can cause the heart muscle to become deprived of oxygen, resulting in heart attack or even sudden death.

Traditional medical doctors treat cardiovascular disease with drugs and surgeries, which are mostly ineffective. One division of the ACCORD trial followed 5518 patients for an average of 4.7 years and found that a combination of two cholesterol-lowering drugs, fenofibrate and Vytorin did not reduce the risk of nonfatal heart attack or stroke, or death from cardiovascular disease in the study population, even though HDL cholesterol increased and triglycerides levels were reduced.[174]

The JUPITER trial showed that lowering LDL cholesterol with drugs showed no benefit.[175] The ENHANCE trial used two cholesterol-lowering medications, and did show that cholesterol was lowered more than when only one drug was used. But the study participants taking the drugs developed more plaque and there was no reduction in the incidence of cardiovascular events.[176]

Angioplasty and bypass surgery do not reduce the risk of adverse cardiovascular events either. The reason is that cardiovascular disease is systemic. If you have vascular disease on one area, you have it everywhere, and these procedures only address plaques in the arteries close to the heart.

There are two types of plaque that form inside the vessel walls; large, calcified plaques and soft, vulnerable plaques. The calcified plaques are not the cause of most heart attacks because they rarely rupture. It is the thousands of soft, vulnerable plaques located in the miles of blood vessels throughout the body that tend to rupture. But the hard, calcified plaques are the ones that are address with procedures.

In 1999, Dr. David Waters of the University of California published the AVERT study in the *New England Journal of Medicine*.[177] Patients in his study were either given Lipitor or were assigned to receive angioplasty with standard follow-up care. The patients who did not receive surgery experienced fewer heart attacks, less chest pain, and made fewer visits to the hospital. According to Dr. Waters, "...atherosclerosis is a systemic disease. It occurs throughout all the coronary arteries. If you fix one segment, a year later it will be another segment that pops and gives you a heart attack, so systemic therapy, with statins or antiplatelet drugs, has the potential to do a lot more."

Even the stent makers have acknowledged that stents do not prevent heart attacks or death. According to Paul LaBiolette, formerly of Boston Scientific, a maker of stents "It's really not about preventing heart attacks, per se; the obvious purpose of the procedure is palliation and symptom relief." [178]

While drugs and surgeries are generally ineffective, the progression of cardiovascular disease can be stopped and it can often even be reversed with diet. Dr. Caldwell Esselstyn at the Cleveland Clinic developed a protocol for treating patients with advanced coronary artery disease, and that have been proven to work in very ill patients, even those who were deemed terminal by their expert cardiologists. He has published articles in medical journals, and has written a book on his scientific findings and his experience treating patients called *Prevent and Reverse Heart Disease.*

In 1985, he began with 24 patients who had collectively experienced 49 cardiovascular events during the eight years prior to the study – 15 cases of angina, 13 cases of measurable disease progression, 7 bypass surgeries, 4 heart attacks, 3 strokes, 2 angioplasties, and 2 worsening stress tests. These were very sick people for whom traditional treatment had failed.

The results were nothing short of spectacular. After dietary intervention:
- Cholesterol was lowered from an average of 246 to well below 150
- Angiograms showed that disease progression had been stopped, and many patients had experienced reversal of the disease
- Angina was improved or eliminated
- Exercise capacity increased, and sexual function was restored
- They required no additional drugs or procedures

6 patients left the study because they thought the diet was too difficult, and here is what happened to them:
- 4 cases of increased angina
- 4 bypass surgeries
- 1 angioplasty
- One case of congestive heart failure
- One death

Only one of the 18 patients remaining in the study experienced worsening health and the reason is that he failed to be compliant with the diet. When he returned to Dr. Esselstyn's eating plan, he experienced improvement again.

11 events in those who dropped out of the study vs. no evens in those who were compliant with the diet. A statistician is not needed to interpret the significance of these results!

As for the claim made by the drop-outs that the diet was hard, I suppose this is a matter of personal perspective. I think chest pain, bypass surgery and death are hard; I'm happy to eat beans and rice and exercise instead!

Dr. Esselstyn has duplicated this success with hundreds of additional patients during the last 24 years, and his work has incredible implications. Heart disease has been the number one killer of Americans for over 100 years.[179] Forty percent of all Americans will die from some form of it.[180] And we spend a fortune treating it - $475 billion per year.[181]

Dr. Esselstyn says, "Heart disease is a toothless paper tiger. It need never exist and if it does, it need never progress."

Erectile Dysfunction

Sex is important to most people, and humans should be able to enjoy it throughout their lives. Unfortunately, more and more men are suffering from erectile dysfunction at earlier and earlier ages. Thirty million men are affected in the U.S. today. Nearly one-third of men in their 50's and more than half in their 60's have this problem. Just watch television for a couple of hours and count the commercials for drugs to treat the condition, and you'll get an idea of how pervasive it has become.

The drug companies have built a billion dollar business around erectile dysfunction. Just one Viagra pill can cost as much as $15. Using it twice a week can cost as much as $1500 per year, and there are no generic versions of the best-selling drugs available yet. In spite of their expense, the drugs don't always work; half of men who take them report that they are ineffective. And there are side effects including stomach discomfort, bladder pain, bloody urine, dizziness, diarrhea, and pain during urination.

Actually, erectile dysfunction really a symptom of cardiovascular disease. Cardiovascular disease causes narrowing arteries as a result of atherosclerotic plaques and damaged endothelial tissue, as you read in the section on heart disease. The body's arteries are not affected regionally; the entire cardiovascular system is damaged by consuming a less-than-optimal diet, and this includes the blood vessels leading to the penis. This is why erectile dysfunction is often the first symptom of cardiovascular disease, and often precedes a heart attack or stroke.[182]

The good news is that by adopting a program of dietary excellence™, beginning an exercise program and losing weight, both cardiovascular disease and erectile dysfunction can be reversed.[183]

Addressing the problem properly through diet and lifestyle has several advantages; it is cheaper than doctor visits and Viagra, there are no negative side effects, and you can reduce the risk of coronary artery disease and all-cause mortality significantly.

The benefits of consuming a well-structured, plant-based diet *are* truly amazing!

Cancer

Just mention cancer in a crowd and the group becomes silent. It's a dreadful disease; difficult to treat; it scares people. And it touches everyone, somehow. It is hard to find a person who has not had cancer, or had a family member or close friend with cancer. Almost all of us have watched cancer patients undergo treatments that sometimes seemed worse than the cancer itself.

The incidence of cancer keeps going up; more and more people are affected. According to the American Cancer Society, American males have a 47% chance of developing cancer and for females the risk is 38%.[184]

Each year, 1,479,350 Americans will be diagnosed with cancer, and 562,340 will die from it –that translates to 1,500 deaths every day![185]

Over-diagnosis is a factor; medical research has shown that aggressive PSA testing and mammography are likely resulting in the diagnosis of many "pseudo-cancers" which really are not cancers requiring treatment, but are treated as cancer anyway.[186] [187] [188] [189] [190] But even after accounting for these inflated statistics, cancer continues to affect more and more people.

The cost of treating cancer is huge - $228.1 billion was spent on cancer treatment in 2009.[191] But we're not getting much return on this investment. Cancer mortality rates have not changed much since Nixon declared the "War on Cancer" in 1971. Yet the cancer industry continues to report that treatments are better and more effective.

For example, a report from the National Center for Health Statistics showed that annual cancer deaths were declining. In 2003, 556,902 people in the U.S. died from cancer, down from 557, 271 the year before.[192] While this is indeed a reduction, it is not even statistically significant – the reduction of only 369 deaths is seven 100ths of a percent. At this rate it will take hundreds of years to cut the death rate from cancer by even 25%.

Even more significant is that most health authorities and organizations continue to insist that cancer is a result of genetic predisposition and environmental factors over which we have no control. They perpetuate the myth that cancer is a mysterious disease of unknown origin that is best treated with surgery and toxic chemicals. But research shows otherwise, as you read earlier.

The most significant contributors to cancer risk are diet and lifestyle. Cancer is not a normal part of aging, nor is its cause unknown. Researchers like Dr. T. Colin Campbell have shown that the right diets can prevent most of the cancers killing large numbers of Americans.

Some people become angry when I talk about the relationship between diet and cancer. They have relatives or friends who have died from cancer and the implication that these people may have been responsible for their illness can be disconcerting. People with cancer often react even more strongly; they sometimes interpret the diet/cancer connection as an accusation that their cancer is "their fault."

I certainly do not intend for my reporting of the scientific facts concerning the cause of cancer to hurt or offend anyone; I want to help people to feel less like victims.
In order to understand the connection between diet and cancer, it is helpful to understand how cancer starts and progresses. Some people think that simple exposure to a carcinogen is all that is required. Fortunately, that it is not the case.

First, carcinogens must be converted to substances that can bind to the DNA of cells and cause mutations. If the body cannot repair a mutated cell prior to cell division, the altered DNA can be passed on to daughter cells, which can be the beginning of cancer.

But these mutated cells will remain dormant until and unless they are acted on by a promoter. Some food components of food are cancer promoters, like animal protein. Others have an anti-cancer effect, like the phytochemicals found in fruits and vegetables. Cancer progresses when there are more cancer promoters than protective nutrients in the diet.

Progression is the phase in which unrestricted growth of cancer cells takes place, and at this time, the cancer may metastasize (move to other sites in the body).

In other words, initiated cancer cells are really not a threat to health until they are acted on by a promoter. Stop consuming cancer promoters, like animal protein, and the opportunity for initiated cells to develop into cancers that are detectable and require treatment is significantly reduced. Dr. Campbell's studies at Cornell showed this to be true. Remember that cancer only developed in the experimental animals when they were fed a diet high in animal protein, and that the cancer started to recede when the animal protein in the diet was lowered to only 5% of calories.[193] In other words the researchers were turning on and turning off cancer in the laboratory based on the percentage of animal protein in the diet.

This should be empowering news for both cancer patients and for people who don't want to get cancer. Instead of feeling helpless, people can significantly reduce their risk of cancer by eating a low-fat, plant-based diet. And there is every reason to believe that diet can positively affect health outcomes for people who have already been diagnosed.

While dietary excellence is important for cancer patients, it is also imperative to have a comprehensive treatment plan. The best resource for evaluating traditional treatments and identifying sometimes much better options is Dr. Ralph Moss at www.cancerdecisions.com. Dr. Moss has developed extensive reports on over 250 types of cancer that provide extensive, life-saving information (the reports are several hundred pages). I know many, many people who would not be alive today had they not consulted with Dr. Moss prior to choosing a treatment plan.

Kay Puldelski's Story

Before I was diagnosed, I felt I was living a glorious life, actually. I was feeling good, and for the most part thinking that I was eating in a very healthy way. I was involved in the fitness industry for about 20 years - so with that background, I felt that I was in control of things and that I was definitely headed for a long and healthy life.

I was surprised when I started seeing some enlarged glands; I thought eventually it would go away, and when it didn't, I saw a doctor. I was diagnosed with Chronic Lymphocytic Leukemia (CLL).

I have a small store, a coffee shop, and I told one of my customers about my situation and he recommended that I read *The China Study*. He also suggested that I talk with another one of our customers, Dr. Pam Popper. I knew Pam, and while I didn't really know anything about her work at the time, I did talk to her.

I read *The China Study,* took Dr. Pam's course, Wellness 101, subscribed to her newsletter, visited her website, and immersed myself in trying to understand what was happening and what to do.

I changed doctors because my first doctor made me feel pretty discouraged; the second one was a little more open-minded. The traditional route for CLL patients is chemotherapy, and sometimes radiation, which I did not want to do. This doctor was willing to let me do my own thing and monitor me. So that was the route I chose – I would change my eating habits and visit the doctor to see how I was doing.

I thought I was eating well but I learned that I was far from it. And so my husband was kind enough to come along with me with the whole new program which really helped. We just emptied the pantry out, emptied the refrigerator, and started anew.

Getting rid of cheese was a big thing for us! It just seemed impossible that anyone could live without it and our refrigerator was full of it. I mean we had drawers of cheese, cans of cheese, you name it. And now, it's all gone.

Grains were not a part of our diet. We had fruit of course, we had vegetables, but not to the degree that we needed. The cookies had to go; I thought that I could not live without them; but they're gone and I do not even think about them anymore. So the pantry and the refrigerator look completely different, in a good way.

Approximately 11 months after I changed my diet, my blood test showed that my counts had gone consistently down and now I am actually at a normal level. Can you believe it? I mean I can't believe it myself! I get teary-eyed thinking about it. But it is normal. My blood cell count is normal.

I would say that the doctor was a bit taken back by the results. He didn't indicate that he was willing to say that diet was the reason the results were what they were. But he could only be pleased for me and was happy with the idea that we would continue to have blood tests done to monitor my health.

I am on board with this diet 100% and so are my husband and my family. It is extending now to my grandchildren. It is really overwhelming, truly overwhelming, and I feel very fortunate.

Diabetes

Diabetes was not common in ancient times, but was a virtual death sentence for anyone who had it, since it was poorly understood and there were no treatments. Insulin was discovered in 1921, which allowed type 1 diabetics to survive. Insulin has also become necessary for many type 2 diabetics because of the progression of their disease.

Diabetes is defined as a condition in which the body either does not produce insulin or is unable to use it properly. Insulin is a hormone produced by the pancreas that helps escort glucose into cells so that it can be used for energy. Type 1 diabetes accounts for approximately five to ten percent of all cases, and results when the insulin–producing cells of the pancreas are destroyed. Although there are many potential causes for destruction of these pancreatic cells, one of the most common is the consumption of cow's milk by infants and children.[194] [195] [196] Patients diagnosed with type 1 diabetes require lifetime treatment with insulin.

Type 2 diabetics produce insulin, but their cells have become insulin-resistant and they are unable to use it. Type-2 diabetes accounts for about 90% of diabetes cases, it is generally considered a byproduct of poor diet and lack of exercise; being overweight is the leading risk factor for developing it.

Gestational diabetes accounts for about two percent of diabetes cases and first appears during pregnancy. Many women with gestational diabetes eventually develop type 2 diabetes. Complications of type 2 diabetes are common and often life–threatening. Diabetics are more likely to develop cardiovascular disease; diabetes is the leading cause of blindness and kidney disease; it accounts for 60% of lower-limb amputations; and many other conditions, including premature death.

During the last several decades, the incidence of diabetes in Westernized countries has been growing at a frightening rate. According to the American Diabetes Association, there are 23.6 million diabetics in the U.S. today; 57 million have pre-diabetes and will develop the condition unless they change their ways.[197]

One of the most frightening trends is the number of children who are developing diabetes. Of new type 2 diabetes cases, 45% are being diagnosed in children.[198]

As a result the condition is no longer referred to as "adult-onset type 2 diabetes," but rather just "type 2 diabetes." Today, 186,300 children under the age of 20 have diabetes in the U.S. and there are two million adolescents between the ages of 12 and 19 who have pre-diabetes. As childhood obesity continues to rise, this number will almost certainly increase. Diabetes is taxing the health care system financially; the cost to treat diabetes *goes up* by an additional $8 billion *every year*![199]

Like other degenerative conditions, diabetes is more prevalent in some areas of the world than in others. Almost 70 years ago, a research report was published comparing different diets and the rate of diabetes in six countries. The study showed that when people eat more carbohydrate and less fat, the number of deaths from diabetes is reduced from 20.4 per 100,000 to 2.9 per 100,000.[200]

But there are variations in the rate of diabetes even within populations in the U.S. Many Seventh Day Adventists do not eat meat, eggs, coffee, or alcohol. About half of them are vegetarian. Almost 90% of Adventists continue to eat foods like eggs and dairy, but overall their consumption of animal foods is considerably lower than that of the average American. Unsurprisingly, Adventists are healthier than most Americans and have half the rate of diabetes of the general population.[201]

Research also shows that Japanese-American men eating the most animal protein, animal fat, and dietary cholesterol are four times more likely to be diabetic than Japanese men living in Japan and eating a more traditional Japanese diet.[202]

Both type 1 and type 2 diabetics benefit from adopting a program of dietary excellence. For type 1 diabetics, the objective is to lower the amount of insulin required and to reduce the incidence of complications, such as cardiovascular disease, neuropathy leading to amputation, retinopathy leading to blindness, and other negative and life-threatening conditions.

Type 2 diabetics almost always get better with dietary improvement and in many cases can expect to reverse their condition, becoming *former* type 2 diabetics.

Dr. James Anderson at the University of Kentucky has conducted studies using dietary intervention on both type 1 and type 2 diabetics. In one study, he placed 25 type 1 and 25 type 2 diabetics on a whole-foods, plant-based diet high in both carbohydrate and fiber. After just three weeks, the type 1 diabetics were able to lower their insulin requirements by 40% and their cholesterol dropped by 30%. Twenty-four out of twenty-five type 2 diabetics were able to *completely discontinue* their insulin medication in only a few weeks.[203]

Dr. Neal Barnard, President of the Physicians' Committee for Responsible Medicine, has also been conducting research using diet to reverse or stop the progression of type 2 diabetes for many years. He has presented his findings at Continuing Medical Education (CME) conferences, published numerous articles in medical journals, and developed an entire division within PCRM to educate diabetics and their families about diet and diabetes.

Dr. Barnard's studies have compared diabetics following a low-fat vegan diet that does not limit the consumption of calories, carbohydrate, or portion sizes, with patients following a diet based on the American Diabetes Association's guidelines. His research consistently shows that patients lose more weight, are able to significantly reduce or even eliminate medications, and show significant improvements in A1C levels (a marker for average blood sugar levels during the previous 2-3 months) after only a few weeks. Additionally, patients following the vegan diet experience rapid drops in blood cholesterol levels, which is significant since most diabetics die from cardiovascular disease.[204] [205]

Diabetes is a highly preventable condition. The risk of type 1 diabetes can be reduced dramatically if parents are instructed not to feed infants and children cow's milk products. Type 2 diabetics can be avoided by practicing dietary excellence and maintaining proper weight and body composition.

But even more important, since millions of people are already diabetic, is the fact that the health of diabetic patients can be dramatically improved with diet and exercise; in fact some people can become *former* diabetics.

Marie Ann Foust's Story

I was always a heavy child. I grew up on a farm and we raised our own animals for meat and eggs, and we had our own dairy cows. My mom was a great cook, and even made her own cottage cheese. Mom always told us to clean our plates and I was happy to comply. I thought these foods were good for me.

Of course, I was an overweight adult, but after my children were born, I started developing other health issues. I had thyroid problems, high cholesterol, high blood pressure, and developed type 2 diabetes. Eventually, I was taking eleven different medications for all the things that were wrong with me. Every time I would visit my doctor, my diseases were worse, or there were more of them; so there were more drugs.

A doctor friend of mine, Dr. Michael Worobiec, cared enough about me to gift me with a membership to The Wellness Forum. I was a little skeptical, but he gave me books to read like *Eat to Live* and *The China Study*. I also watched lots of DVD lectures from doctors who use diet to help their patients. I became really excited that I might be able to stop taking some of my medications. I started changing my diet right away.

Today, just a few short months later, I am a *former* diabetic who has lost 53 pounds. I now only take three drugs. I just had a blood test done and for the first time in my life, my numbers are normal. I do aerobic exercise every day, and I've started walking – I'm up to 2 miles now.

My biggest challenge is getting used to some of the new foods. I love vegetables, but I'm still not wild about tofu. I've taken classes with Chef Del, and I'm learning how to season food without salt and appreciate new tastes.

I cannot say enough about good things about The Wellness Forum and also the great support I've had from Dr. Worobiec.

To lose weight was a dream; to get healthy and stop taking so many of these drugs was just amazing!

Autoimmune Diseases

Although there are over forty different autoimmune diseases that affect people in many diverse ways, these diseases all follow the same pattern; the immune system mistakenly attacks the body's cells. In the case of type 1 diabetes, the target is the pancreatic cells that produce insulin; for multiple sclerosis it is the myelin sheath that protects the nerves; and in Graves Disease it is the thyroid gland. The common denominator of all autoimmune diseases is the loss of the body's ability to differentiate "self" from "non-self."

The immune system is designed to protect our bodies against foreign invaders by producing cells that attack viruses and bacteria that appear in the body as protein molecules called antigens.

When antigens appear, the immune system responds by creating a similar protein called an antibody, which attacks and neutralizes the antigen. The immune system creates a different antibody for each antigen. Once the antibody is created, it is used every time that particular antigen appears in the body. Thus your immune system's "memory" can keep you from getting sick when an antigen reappears, even after a long absence. This is the case with flu viruses, for example. An initial exposure to a new strain of flu might make you ill; but the body may be able to deal with future exposures to the same virus *before* it can make you sick. You may not even be aware that your body has even encountered the virus again.

People develop autoimmune diseases when immune cells begin attacking the very tissues they are designed to protect. Medical professionals hypothesize about many causes for these conditions, including viruses and lack of sunlight. But a growing body of research points to "molecular mimicry" as the cause of many autoimmune diseases.

Some of the amino acids chains making up the antigens that our immune cells attack look remarkably like some of the amino acid chains that make up our tissues and organs. In most cases, our bodies are able to differentiate a foreign invader from our own tissues. But in some instances, the antibodies created to attack

216

those antigens will begin attacking our own cells which have a similar appearance.

As it turns out, some of those antigens that "fool" the body into attacking its own cells are in the foods we eat. During the process of digestion, it is not uncommon for some proteins to move from the intestines into the bloodstream without being fully broken down. These undigested proteins are perceived as foreign invaders and treated as such; the immune system mobilizes and manufactures antibodies to attack them. Those antibodies sometimes then mistakenly attack tissues and organs that look like the original antigen.

For example, undigested cow's milk protein fragments look very similar to the pancreatic cells that produce insulin. When the immune system cannot differentiate between proteins from cow's milk and pancreatic cells, it begins attacking and destroying pancreatic cells, which reduces or stops the production of insulin. Studies have shown a relationship between the consumption of cow's milk and the incidence of type 1 diabetes in many countries.[206]

The relationship between diet and autoimmune diseases is not limited to type 1 diabetes. Like many other conditions, there seems to be a correlation between the consumption of a Westernized diet concentrated in animal foods and the incidence of autoimmune diseases. But it appears that just as a poor diet can contribute to the development of autoimmune diseases, an optimal one can stop the progression of or reverse them.

Lynne Synatschk's Story

I was called "the meat and potatoes" girl by my family while growing up, and I continued to eat that way as an adult. Unfortunately, my family followed in my footsteps too. We all drank soft drinks instead of water; ate meat instead of vegetables; and about the only good food we had with any degree of regularity was fruit.

In 1997, I experienced a mysterious pain in my arm that quickly spread throughout my body until I literally hurt from head to toe. About six months later I was diagnosed with fibromyalgia. I was determined to avoid taking drugs, so I started doing some research and determined that dietary supplements and high-dose vitamins would help to make things better. I took them, but I didn't get better.

A couple of years later, my health had gotten even worse, and I was diagnosed with lupus. A friend suggested that maybe the problem was my diet. I still didn't want to take drugs, so I thought I'd look into it, and I started learning a little bit about whole food nutrition. I got rid of the soft drinks and we started drinking water, and I served salads with every meal. My kids were furious, but the more I learned, the more convinced I became that diet was important.

Through a friend, I found out about Dr. Pam Popper, and during my first conversation with her I asked her if she thought I could reverse my lupus naturally and she said yes. This was the first ray of hope I had in a long, long time. I immediately started changing my diet, and really my entire life at that point. I read not only Dr. Popper's books, but books written by Dr. Esselstyn, Dr. McDougall and others who reinforced the idea that diet could make me well.

I started feeling better, but my blood tests still showed high ANA levels (antibodies that indicate lupus). After a while, I decided that the blood tests were just making me upset, so I decided to stop visiting my doctor. I was lucky, in that he did not try to push me into taking drugs, but I could not afford to have anything interfere with my mental attitude in getting well.

I was able to regain most of my health by eating a plant-based diet, but the final piece in my recovery was a trip to TrueNorth to do a water-only fast. That was a remarkable experience; I lost weight, and my allergies, which had already gotten better, completely went away. My diet improved even more; giving up high-fat vegetarian foods and oils made a big difference.

In March 2008, I worked up enough courage to go to my doctor for a blood test. I was shocked when I was told that my ANA levels had returned to normal. I was so excited and I could not wait to tell Dr. Popper that I was now a *former* lupus patient!

Today, my whole life is different. When I had lupus, I was tired, my joints were stiff, I had irritable bowel syndrome, and I could not sleep. Now, those things are not an issue, and my brain is not foggy any more either. I have lots of energy, which allows me to do everything I want to do, which includes enjoying and keeping up with my grandson!

Multiple Sclerosis

Multiple sclerosis (MS) is an autoimmune disease that affects the central nervous system. In the case of MS, the immune system destroys the insulating sheath that covers the nerve fibers. This then interferes with the body's ability to send messages to and from the brain and spinal cord.

MS is generally diagnosed between the ages of 20 and 40 and women are three times more likely to develop it than men.[207] It is a highly unpredictable condition and can present in a number of different ways. The most common form is referred to as "relapsing-remitting" which involves episodes referred to as exacerbations followed by remissions. The disease continues to progress, however, and often leads to disability. Another form is called "primary-progressive," which means the disease consistently progresses from the onset. MS may later progress after a period of relapsing and remitting, which is referred to as secondary progression. Regardless of the pattern, MS patients do not fare well. Within 10 years, 50% of all MS patients are either walking with assistance, confined to a wheelchair or deceased.

Symptoms of MS include numbness and tingling in the extremities; optic neuritis; weakness, spasm and paraplegia; difficulties in walking; bladder or bowel dysfunction; pain; fatigue; and cognitive difficulty.

The late Dr. Roy Swank headed the Division of Neurology at the University of Oregon Medical School and became interested in the connection between diet and MS after observing that the condition seemed to be more prevalent in northern climates. Dr. Swank theorized that the reason might be that people living further away from the equator were consuming diets that included more animal foods and were higher in saturated fats.

Dr. Swank tested his theory on 144 MS patients, who were told to consume a diet low in saturated fat. He followed this group for 34 years, and tracked the progression of their disease.[208]

Some of Dr. Swank's patients were compliant and others were not. He categorized his patients based on their fat consumption

– "good dieters" consumed less than 20 grams per day of saturated fat; "bad dieters" consumed more than 20 grams per day. Patients in the group consuming less than 20 grams of fat per day fared significantly better than the group eating more fat. For those who ate a low-saturated fat diet, "about 95%...remained only mildly disabled for approximately 30 years." Eighty-percent of the patients who consumed more saturated fat died of MS.[209] Dr. Swank published several articles in medical journals documenting his results.[210] [211] [212]

After Dr. Swank began his research, studies showed a connection between multiple sclerosis and cow's milk. This link was confirmed in a study of populations in twenty four countries that showed a clear connection between consuming cow's milk and the incidence of MS.[213] Dr. Swank and others proved that two staples of the Standard American Diet, dairy and saturated fat, increased the risk of MS.

Medications used to treat MS are highly toxic and do little to stop the progression of the condition. The Cochrane Collaboration is a non-profit organization that conducts research on many medical issues, including the safety and efficacy of drugs. According to Cochrane Collaboration reviews on drugs commonly used to treat MS (Copaxone, Interferon and Corticosteroids), they are effective for relieving symptoms, but do not provide long-term benefit, and in some cases their side effects and costs outweigh any potential benefit.[214] [215] [216] Dietary intervention, on the other hand, almost always results in improvement, has no negative side effects, and is inexpensive.

Dr. John McDougall has been successfully treating MS patients with a low-fat, plant-based diet for many years. Dr. McDougall's approach is based on Dr. Swank's research, but his diet is even lower in fat, calls for the elimination of both dairy products and oils, and does not include dietary supplements. After adopting his diet, his MS patients are generally drug-free and most live normal lives, without symptoms.

The response from other medical doctors about using diet instead of drugs has been less than enthusiastic, with many insisting that randomized controlled studies have not proven the value of the diet. Determined to overcome this criticism, Dr.

McDougall has raised $750,000 to fund a randomized controlled trial that will prove to the medical community using MRI scans and disability evaluations that a low-fat plant-based diet works to stop the progression of or even reverse MS. This is an extraordinary commitment of both money and time, and has the potential to benefit tens of thousands of people.

I asked Dr. McDougall why he chose to do a study on Multiple Sclerosis patients, and he replied that MS is such a horrific disease and so hard to treat; he believes that if he can show that diet works for this condition, he can convince people that it will work for many others as well.

Christine Smothers' Story

I'm a personal trainer and athlete; for a long time I did competitive body building. I looked great while I was competing, but had no idea that I was destroying my body. I think sometimes people just assume athletes are in optimal health, but I learned the hard way that this is not always the case.

In my early 20's my diet and lifestyle were anything but healthy – I smoked, drank Dr. Pepper for energy, and ate generally unhealthy foods.

Eventually, I started running and it seemed a little weird to smoke after running, so I decided to quit, which was really very hard – more so emotionally than physically. People told me I needed to replace my smoking habit with something else, so I decided to replace it with fitness. I loved the "high" I got from running, and it was even better after I quit smoking. I started thinking that I'd like to help other people with their health and fitness, so I became a fitness trainer. While getting certified, I met some people who were into competitive body building. I found that body building also gave me the "high" that running did, so I pursued that too.

The trainers I worked with gave me what I thought was good diet advice – they had been in the field for many years and I trusted them. They told me that if I wanted to compete and win, I needed to eat a very high protein diet, with minimal fat and carbohydrate. I did what they told me to do – I ate egg whites for breakfast, chicken and salad for snacks, and fish and salads for lunch and dinner. I also ate a lot of whey protein in the form of sports drinks. My meals were all centered around animal protein.

I looked great, but to be honest, I felt bad more than I felt good. I was sick, tired, and irritable all the time. In fact, people did not want to be around me when I was competing because this was when my diet was the most extreme and I felt the worst.

Eventually I decided to go back to school to finish my degree in athletic training and I stopped competing to make time for that. But I continued to eat the same diet since I was used to it and I thought it was healthy.

The real problems started with flu-like symptoms that just didn't seem to get better. Then I started having episodes of severe pain, numbness, tingling, and even paralysis. This really frightened me – I would feel fine and all of a sudden have an "attack" and I couldn't move.

I spoke to a physician colleague at school who told me he thought I had multiple sclerosis. I was in denial, but after another episode, I couldn't ignore what was happening any more, so I went to my family doctor. I spent five days in a hospital hoping the doctors would tell me this was anything but MS, but left with a firm diagnosis. And I left with drugs; drugs for depression, anxiety, pain, and Interferon to control the MS symptoms.

I took the drugs like I was supposed to for five months, and then started becoming concerned about the side effects. I also started thinking about Dr. Pam Popper – I had met her about 12 years before all of this. I remembered the things she said about diet and health, so I decided to contact her.

By the time we met, I was ready to get off the drugs and change my diet. I started the plant-based diet immediately and I got better. In fact, a lot better. I was so excited and felt so good that I decided I wanted to do something to help other people with MS. There are a lot of organizations that are trying to help MS patients, but they really promote drug treatment, not diet and lifestyle.

I had learned about Dr. John McDougall from Dr. Popper, and knew that he also used diet to treat MS, and was raising money to conduct a study. So I decided to raise money for Dr. McDougall by doing a bike tour. Although I had never cycled before, I wanted to try it and it would allow me to see parts of the U.S. I had never seen before. There was another important reason too. Many of the people I know are victimized by their diseases; they are unable to do lots of things. I didn't want to be that way; I wanted to prove to myself and others that I was not limited by my diagnosis.

MS patients usually cannot tolerate heat. I took hot yoga classes in a 105 degree room and did fine. MS patients usually have trouble with exertion. Well, riding over 300 miles to Canada would prove that this did not apply to me either.

So I recruited a team of family and friends who were into cycling, I approached Dr. McDougall to get his blessing, and we did it! We rode 80-100 miles per day for three and a half days. I did all but 20 miles of it – that had nothing to do with my MS, but I had a knee injury that briefly caused me some problems.

We raised $2000 for Dr. McDougall and I have to say this was the most rewarding thing I ever did other than giving birth to my son.

And this brings me to the most important thing of all. My son used to be like other kids – he ate bad foods, he was overweight and he sat in front of a computer instead of exercising. I tried to tell him to eat better and exercise, but looking back, I was preaching, not teaching.

When I got sick, I decided my son and I were going to get healthier together. We both attended the Wellness Forum classes offered at Dr. Popper's office and he started changing his diet too. Today, he is normal weight and eats a plant-based diet like I do, even at college! What I went through was frightening, but the great byproduct of my experience has been my son's health improvement and weight loss.

I learned the hard way how important it is to stay compliant on the diet. The only relapse I've had was a result of letting some things creep into my diet that I should not have eaten. I clearly see the connection between what I eat and my health now.

I'm so much better off than MS patients who are taking drugs. I've learned that a frightening diagnosis does not have to be a life sentence. You can overcome many things and change the direction of your life. I am not going to be another MS statistic.

Gastrointestinal Disorders

During the last several decades, Americans have become quite preoccupied with the discomfort of digestion. Digestion is a normal process whereby food is converted into substances that enter the bloodstream and are delivered to the cells to be utilized for energy and function. The waste byproducts of digestion are eliminated in the feces.

Healthy people are generally not even aware that their bodies are digesting food. Unhealthy people, on the other hand, often experience discomfort and even pain as a result of digestion and elimination. Gall bladder disease, reflux, bloating, indigestion, diarrhea, constipation, and other gastrointestinal disorders have become very common, and the drug companies are making a fortune marketing drugs to relieve symptoms of these very uncomfortable conditions. Tens of millions of Americans suffer from constipation and hundreds of millions of dollars are spent on laxatives alone every year.

In addition to discomfort and pain, digestive disorders contribute to the development of other issues such as halitosis (bad breath), skin conditions like eczema and psoriasis, iron deficiency, nutrient deficiencies, allergies, and bone loss.

There are many causes of gastrointestinal disorders, but the main causes are taking drugs like antibiotics, and diets rich in meat, dairy, fat, and refined foods.

One of the byproducts of certain drugs and poor diet is destruction of beneficial bacteria in the GI tract. The friendly bacteria in the GI tract are important to health. There are hundreds of different strains of friendly bacteria, which exist in several pounds of partially digested organic material in the intestinal tract. These bacteria assist in many functions including digesting food, synthesizing water-soluble vitamins, and stimulating immune function. They also prevent overgrowth of pathogenic bacteria.[217]

Beneficial bacteria grow and colonize best on a diet that includes lots of plant foods, since their preferred nutrient is carbohydrate.

Pathogenic bacteria such as parasites and yeasts prefer the residue from animal foods.

Adopting a program of dietary excellence™ can increase the population of friendly bacteria and decrease the population of unfriendly bacteria, and studies show that this effect begins within only a couple of weeks after positive dietary change.[218]

Conditions like constipation, bloating and reflux are uncomfortable, but far more serious GI disorders are becoming increasingly common. The most severe are called inflammatory bowel disease (IBD). There are two main types – ulcerative colitis and Crohn's disease, which affect different parts of the intestinal tract. Symptoms include pain in the abdomen, bloody diarrhea, and mucus. Many patients have 20 or more bloody, mucus-filled, and loose bowel movements per day; it is not uncommon for these patients' lives to revolve around being near a bathroom at all times. Obviously, these conditions adversely affect quality of life for the patients who suffer from them. They are of great concern because patients suffering from IBD are at higher risk of developing colon cancer.
Inflammatory bowel diseases result from consuming dairy products, animal fat and protein, and refined and processed foods.[219]

Fat in the diet is a major contributor to IBD, which is more common in areas where people consume a Western diet. One study involving U.S. patients in Japan showed that those who consumed higher fat diets were 2.5 times more likely to develop IBD – even if the fats were those referred to by some as "good fats," like vegetable oils and Omega-3 fatty acids.[220]

Sulfur-containing amino acids in animal foods interact with bacteria in the bowel, creating sulfur compounds that increase inflammation and exacerbating symptoms.[221]

Cow's milk is another food that increases the risk of IBD;[222] other common triggers include high-gluten foods, high-sugar and refined foods. [223]

Traditional treatments include immunosuppressant drugs and surgery to remove parts of the bowel that are inflamed. These treatments do not stop the progression of the disease, however, and patients continue to get worse.

Adopting a well-structured plant-based diet with the exclusion of trigger foods is effective for treating IBD.[224] One study showed that two-thirds of the patients who were treated with improved diet were well two years after converting to a healthier diet.[225]

In addition to dietary change, the balance of friendly and unfriendly bacteria is usually so impaired that probiotics are required to restore intestinal health. Probiotic products are comprised of several strains of friendly bacteria, and although they can be purchased in health food stores, the best and strongest ones are available through licensed doctors. Consumed orally, these products assist in re-establishing the proper balance of bacteria in the GI tract, which helps restore normal function.

Liz Kuhn's Story

I developed Crohn's disease when I was 25. At the time I was suffering from a really bad bout of diarrhea that had gone on for several months. I had lost quite a bit of weight, was fatigued all the time, and eating was not a pleasant experience for me, so I tried to cut that out as much as I possibly could. Sleeping was very difficult because I was up many times during the night. It was very difficult to continue working a full-time job at that time. I was under a great deal of stress, in the process of going through a divorce, so it was a very stressful time all the way around.

I saw a gastroenterologist that I continued to see for 25 years; I developed a very good relationship with him. He placed me on a course of steroids and drugs that I took for the majority of the next 15 years. For the most part I would have a flare-up every three years; I would end up in the hospital for a couple of weeks with bleeding and hemorrhaging episodes. I'd be off work for two to four weeks at a time. I was very lucky I never had to have surgery; I came extremely close on a number of occasions, but was always able to avoid it.

The fatigue was really the hardest; I was not absorbing any nutrients from the foods that I was eating so life was very, very difficult.

During the time I was sick, I was told to stay away from vegetables. Vegetables and fruit were the hardest on my system, so I stuck pretty much to meat and potatoes; rice was not recommended at all. I ate a lot of sweets and bread because I thought they were the blandest things I could possibly eat. I did realize at that time that dairy was not a good thing for me, so dairy got cut out pretty much at the very beginning of the diagnosis.

I ate pretty much everything that was bad for me; all the sweets and cakes and cookies and things that I loved. Combined with taking steroids, I was gaining a lot of weight unless I was having a flare-up (I tried not to eat during those times). At one point at 5'7", my weight was up to almost 200 pounds.

The last flare-up I had, interesting enough, was September 11, 2001. Everybody knows where they were on that day; I was in the hospital. I had started hemorrhaging at work and was raced to the emergency room.

The doctors recommended a course of treatment that included Remicade infusions. It worked and the Crohn's went away; it was kept under control. But the side effects of being on an immune suppressant drug were severe: I developed pneumonia twice; I started having abnormal pap smears; I developed huge cysts in my breasts; and the kicker was that they found a spot on my lungs at the end of that first year.

By this time, I had started a working relationship with Dr. Pam Popper and I told her what was going on. When the spot on my lungs was detected, that really frightened me and at that time I decided I needed to get off my medications.

I talked to my gastroenterologist and he agreed that it was worth trying. So I quit all my medications cold turkey. I started working with Dr. Pam on changing my diet. My new diet eliminated all products that contained gluten, and dairy products. She also recommended that I give up sugar, and I've been about 75% good with that, but you know chocolate *is* chocolate.

It has been tough on occasion. I love bread. I love noodles. I love sweets. But I have learned to put it in perspective and realize that I would rather be healthy. And a lot of food that I eat now tastes just as great. It's just something different. And raw fruits and raw vegetables, which would have been unheard of when I was thirty, are the major portion of what I eat now. And I am trying to branch out to try some new things. I have learned to find gluten-free pastas and other products too.

I am not a complete vegetarian or a vegan. I still love my steak. But where I was having meat up to four times a week, now I have meat once every six months and the majority is turkey. I still do love seafood; that I have a little more often.

Combining my new eating habits with exercise on a regular basis, I dropped 50 pounds. I am probably in the best shape that I have ever been in my life. I do fitness boxing; I am learning to ride a motorcycle; I have gone parasailing and waterskiing and snow skiing; all sorts of different adventures. It has just been a wonderful experience not being restricted by needing to be close to a bathroom and worrying about when I am going to get sick.

My energy level is a lot better, I am a lot more active, and I keep busy doing other things. When I was fighting Crohn's, a big night for me was going out to the movies. I didn't go out with my friends - I basically worked, came home, and either tried to get some sleep or watched television. And now I am out meeting friends to do various activities. I have my own website design business and that keeps me very busy. I am very active in my church and church activities. So my life has just blossomed. Like I said I am into adventures and trying new things so it has just been a wonderful, wonderful blessing, in finding Dr. Pam and the Wellness Forum program. And I truly feel like I have conquered Crohn's disease.

I did go back to see my gastroenterologist, at my four-year anniversary of being totally off all medications. He told me at that time that he was shocked and he had fully expected me to be back within the first couple of months asking for my medications back. The fact that I had gone four years, he said he had never seen positive results like that. So he was totally impressed.

Infertility and Miscarriage

Infertility is becoming a major health issue in the U.S. According to the American Pregnancy Association, 6,000,000 American women are experiencing infertility,[226] about 10% of women of reproductive age. According to a 2005 Centers for Disease Control report,[227] 134,260 in vitro fertilization procedures were reported to the agency, more than double the rate of less than a decade ago. It is estimated that 15% of all couples have to deal with fertility issues at some time in their lives.

In addition to the stress inflicted on couples who are unable to conceive, the financial cost is incredible. In vitro fertilization is the most successful medical treatment used to remedy infertility. The cost for a single cycle of in vitro fertilization is between $7000 and $11,000. Additionally, medications average $1500 per cycle. Only 42% of these procedures result in a pregnancy, and 35% result in a live birth.[228] There are only four states that mandate insurance coverage for these procedures, so most of the time they are paid for by the patient.

There are numerous causes for infertility and some of them require medical intervention. But much of the time, the cause is related to diet and lifestyle. The same hormone imbalances that have caused millions of women to experience PMS, cramping, dysmenorrhea, and horrible menopausal symptoms are often the cause of infertility, too.

A study published in the November 2007 issue of *Obstetrics and Gynecology* showed that women consuming more monounsaturated fats instead of trans fats, vegetable protein instead of animal protein, increased fiber, and low glycemic carbohydrates had improved fertility outcomes.

"Our results suggest that a fertility diet pattern may have favorable effects on the fertility of otherwise healthy women and that combining this dietary strategy with body weight control and increased physical activity may help prevent the majority of infertility cases due to problems with ovulation," the study authors concluded. [229]

Another study looked at the effects of animal protein on fertility; 18,555 married women with a history of infertility were followed for eight years. The 20% of the women who ate the highest amount of animal protein had a 39% increased risk of ovulatory infertility. The researchers concluded "replacing animal sources of protein with vegetable sources of protein may reduce ovulatory infertility risk."[230]

Women who consume low-fat dairy products may be at increased risk of infertility. Researchers reported that two or more servings of low-fat dairy daily increased the risk of infertility by 85%.[231]

The high cost of fertility treatments, combined with their low success rates make dietary improvement a better option in many cases. Women were specifically designed and engineered to conceive, carry and give birth to children, but are much more likely to be able to do so when they are in optimal health.

Molly Wallace's Story

Four years ago my husband I started talking about having a family. You never think you are going to have difficulties in this area, but looking back, I had very irregular cycles and that was my first hint that I might have challenges down the road.

About six months after we decided to take the plunge, I still was not pregnant, and we were getting concerned. I visited my ob/gyn, who told me that it was not unusual for it to take up to a year to conceive. We continued to try and I did get pregnant, but had a miscarriage. It was a very difficult and devastating experience.

I ended up having two more miscarriages – a total of three in about a year. By that time, the doctors were concerned; they consider three miscarriages a sign of significant infertility.

During this time, no one talked to me about diet at all. But I decided to do my own homework because that is the type of person I am. I researched as much as I could about infertility and miscarriages and I did find some things that indicated diet and lifestyle were important. But when I brought it up to a reproductive endocrinologist he looked me right in the eye and told me that diet had nothing to do with my problem. My husband was sitting right there and heard it too.

The endocrinologist wanted us to begin IVF (in vitro fertilization) treatment. That was the first suggestion he made, even before we had a conversation. I wanted to get to the root cause of these miscarriages. I was not ready for that step, so we didn't do it.

Shortly after this conversation, I mentioned to him that based on my research, I might be experiencing some insulin resistance. He didn't agree but I pleaded with him to run some tests and sure enough, I did show some signs of insulin resistance. This did not surprise me since diabetes runs in my family.

At this point I was really discouraged. I felt like I needed a good team of people who could guide me. I did not know where to turn – I thought the nutrition piece was key, but no one wanted to talk to me about it.

I was frustrated, and after three miscarriages I decided I did not want to put my body through any more. And I needed an emotional break, too. I started thinking about how we were approaching getting pregnant; the more I thought about fertility treatments and drugs the more I was convinced I wanted a more natural approach.

I had heard about Dr. Pam Popper through a friend and recommended that my mother see her because she had an autoimmune disease. One day when I was talking to my mom, she said that she had had such good results with Dr. Pam she could not understand why I hadn't called her myself. I thought to myself, "that's right!" And I made an appointment right away.

Right after I talked to Dr. Pam, my husband and I took a vacation, and I had the Wellness 101 book on the plane. I kept interrupting him to tell him the things I was learning. He really got that this was something important to me, and he ended up reading the book and jumping on board with me.

At this time, I was excited because I felt like "Aha! I have the answer!" I felt empowered; I was getting some control back, and I had a plan.

Within a couple of months, my body started to change. All the puffiness in my face, acne, and belly fat – it all went away. I felt like a new person. I started to think that what I was trying to do was to create a healthy home for this baby that would be coming soon. I was thinking positively again and I could visualize having a baby and my dream coming true.

I was still a little nervous about getting pregnant but after a few months, my cycles were becoming normal and I thought my body was ready. We got pregnant in April – six months after I saw Dr. Pam, and had a very healthy pregnancy. We were very blessed and everything went perfectly.

Being a mom is better than I could even imagine. Things happen for a reason. When I made the shift from "if" to "when" we would have a family, I started thinking about how much healthier our whole family was going to be because of the things I went through that resulted in my new diet and lifestyle.

The pediatrician says my son Ben is the picture of health!

Nancy Mesko's Story

I was raised on a dairy farm like Dr. Campbell and many others, so I grew up on a very rich diet of all the milk I wanted. We had 10,000 laying hens so I had access to as many eggs as I wanted too. And obviously lots of meat. We ate lots of fruits and vegetables but had a very meat-heavy diet. As an adult, I really cut back on red meat, but ate lots of chicken, turkey, fish, low-fat dairy products, and low-fat processed foods. I thought I was eating really well since everything was lower in fat. Everyone thought I was the picture of health. I was very active, I exercised.

I took birth control pills for 3 or 4 years, and my medical problems started when I decided to stop taking them. Immediately I stopped having menstrual cycles. My OB/GYN assured me that this was quite normal, and eventually would fix itself. After over a year, nothing changed and I was diagnosed with polycystic ovary disease. I was advised to take fertility drugs if I wanted my cycles to start again, but that didn't seem like a good idea to me.

I continued to go to doctors and over the years I was diagnosed with Graves Disease, osteopenia, and eventually at the age of 35 was told that I was becoming menopausal. I was really concerned about that, but the doctors told me this was really normal and becoming more common all the time.

By this time, I was really concerned about my health, so I did a little research on my own and started eating more of a whole foods diet. Shortly after, I met Dr. Pam Popper. Although I was already eating better, I cleaned my diet up even more based on her recommendations. Within only a few months, I started having menstrual cycles again after 3 ½ years of not having them. About 18 months later, I had another bone density test done, and the osteopenia had completely reversed itself.
I was married for 10 years and tried without success to get pregnant, and was menopausal at 35, so I really never expected to have children. But six years from the time I started changing my diet, I became pregnant at the age of 41. My baby was born on the due date at 8 pounds 6 ounces only 20 minutes after I got to the hospital. I feel so blessed not only to have this child, but to be able to help him start out in life with the right diet.

Other members of my family have benefited from plant-based nutrition too. My dad had a heart attack, and after that I was able to get him to change his eating habits. He's not an "A" student, but he does understand the value of eating plant-based. I know that's the only reason he is still with us today.

I look back and I am so grateful for people like Dr. Popper, Dr. Campbell and Dr. Barnard that have really stepped outside of the traditional medical model and have been there for people like me!

Asthma

Twenty million Americans suffer from asthma,[232] and according to the Asthma and Allergy Foundation of America, half of those cases are "allergic-asthma." Asthma is the most common chronic condition in children.[233] [234]

Each year, $18 billion is spent treating asthma, and it is the number one illness that keeps kids out of school,[235] causing them to miss 14 million school days each year. There are more hospitalizations due to asthma than any other childhood illness, and kids spend eight million days in bed each year as a result of it.[236]

Asthma is a chronic respiratory disease involving inflammation and obstruction of the airways. Its symptoms include shortness of breath, tightness in the chest and coughing. Because of the recent rapid increase in the incidence of asthma, many people assume that its causes are environmental, from factors like air pollution and chemical exposure.

But asthma is more prevalent in developed countries; in less developed countries where the pollution rates are often much higher, the incidence of asthma is generally a lot lower. Although air pollution has been shown to exacerbate symptoms of asthma, it has never been proven to cause it. [237] [238]

It's not the environment that is causing this epidemic; it's diet. Dairy products are particularly common allergens and contribute to asthmatic symptoms.[239] [240]

Another factor that contributes to asthma is acid reflux, which is also related to diet. [241] [242] Reflux is common in people who are overweight and/or who consume the rich Western diet. This causes weakness in the esophageal sphincter, which allows tiny amounts of acid to leak into the esophageal tube. In addition to causing extreme discomfort and even pain, the acid travels to the back of the throat. As the acid is inhaled, the bronchial tubes are burned. The body attempts to reduce the inflammation by increasing production of mucus, inducing symptoms of asthma.

Asthma is commonly treated with steroids and other drugs; many patients carry inhalers for emergency situations when they simply cannot breathe. But there are serious concerns with some of the drugs used to treat it. A meta-analysis of 19 trials involving 36,826 asthma patients found that commonly used drugs like Serevent increase the incidence of hospitalizations related to asthma and asthma-related deaths.[243]

Since asthma is diet-induced and pharmaceutical treatments are risky, the best strategy for treating it is to adopt a well-structured plant-based diet. Research shows that dietary improvement can reduce the need for medications and the frequency and severity of asthma attacks.[244] Asthmatics who are compliant with their diets and maintain optimal weight should be able to lead a normal life without the use of drugs. Many become *former* asthma patients.

Henry Hageman's Story

I grew up near a large dairy farm, and I drank more milk than water. My mom was a heavy smoker. Looking back, it's not surprising that my health issues started almost from birth. I had raging eczema until I was two, which was replaced with horrific asthma.

My asthma worsened, and eventually I developed allergies and chronic staph infections. In spite of taking lots of drugs for these conditions, I routinely missed school for as long as two weeks at a time.

Every year in March as Spring approached, my allergies would get worse. I had to carry at least one box of Kleenex with me everywhere I went. Shortly after the first frost, the asthma would return, and I'd start to get colds regularly, all of which would almost immediately go into my chest.

As if all of that was not enough, as an adult I suffered from low blood sugar, which would cause my energy levels to drop rapidly. My solution for that was to go to the nearest fast food restaurant and eat lots of food – sometimes three sandwiches or three orders of French fries at a time. I ate my way into a real weight problem. I was able to keep going mainly because of coffee – my habit peaked at 17 cups per day.

It's almost amazing to me but the person who inspired me to change my diet was an oncologist. My dad had heart disease, my mother was recovering from a stroke and my father-in-law was diagnosed with bone cancer. His oncologist told my wife and me that it was too late for my father-in-law, but that we could both escape our family history by changing our diets and eating more fruits and vegetables. He pointed out research that showed that populations that ate the most produce had the lowest rates of chronic disease.

We immediately changed our ways, bought a juicer, and things started getting better. We were inspired to do more, and eventually converted to a plant-based diet, giving up dairy foods and meat. It was like a lightning bolt when I started eating real whole foods! The allergies were so much better, I wasn't tired. I stopped taking my blood pressure medication, and lost 70 pounds. Eventually I did not need an inhaler anymore.

I always loved running, but there were some days when I was so congested that I just could not do it. On better days, I'd try to run and took my inhaler with me, but I often could not finish my run. Today I can run whenever I like, and I've completed two marathons.

I feel great, look great, and love life on this plant-based diet. I know my wife and I have reduced the risk of the diseases that plagued our parents, and can look forward to a longer and better life.

Arthritis

Arthritis and joint pain are so common that many people consider them a normal part of aging. But they are not – healthy people do not experience arthritis pain, and joints are designed to last and function for an entire lifetime!

There are several types of arthritis, but most people have either osteoarthritis or some form of inflammatory arthritis. Joint pain can be a symptom of arthritis or caused by poor diet, lack of exercise and being overweight.

Osteoarthritis is a degenerative condition that results from poor diet and lifestyle choices. People who consume a Western-style diet with lots of animal protein, fat, and processed foods are more likely to be overweight or obese, which places undue stress on the hips, knees, and joints, causing pain and eventually damage. Consumption of excess fat impairs circulation to the all of the joints, including the fingers, elbows, and shoulders, depriving them of necessary nutrients and fluids. Lack of exercise can exacerbate joint pain since movement is needed in order for synovial fluid to be released from cartilage which helps keep joints lubricated.

Inflammatory arthritic conditions include rheumatoid arthritis, lupus, and ankylosing spondylitis. Animal foods are rich in arachadonic acid, which can cause inflammation, and the over-consumption of meat and dairy foods can cause increased production of inflammatory hormones. Fat cells produce inflammatory cytokines, which makes excess body fat an independent risk factor for arthritis.

Gout is a form of inflammatory arthritis experienced mostly by men, and is a result of the accumulation of uric acid crystals; the big toe is the most commonly affected joint. Gout is also a direct result of consuming a diet high in animal protein and fat.

People with arthritis often have pain that can be incredibly crippling and intolerable; pain medication is sometimes needed in order for patients to function. Pain medications do not address the underlying condition; they all have unpleasant and sometimes health-destroying side effects; patients often build a tolerance to the drugs, necessitating the use of even stronger drugs, and some are addictive.

Conversion to a well-structured plant-based diet causes fast relief from arthritis pain because the diet reduces consumption of foods that contribute to inflammation. It also results in weight loss, which reduces pressure on the lower extremities, and the production of inflammatory cytokines from fat cells. Most early-stage arthritis patients will recover fully with dietary change, weight loss, and exercise. Some of the deformity and damage to joints and cartilage from many years of abuse cannot be reversed, but pain can be relieved, the progression of the disease can be stopped, and disability can be avoided. A proper exercise program can help patients to re-gain both strength and range of motion; yoga is particularly helpful for arthritis patients.

Rose Byrd's Story

I learned about the Wellness Forum and Dr. Pam Popper at about the same time I was being diagnosed with rheumatoid arthritis. At that time I was having pain in my hands, and my arms and my hands were swelling. Sometimes I could barely move my fingers, and a couple of times I couldn't even get dressed for work.

I went to my family doctor, who referred me to an arthritis center where I was diagnosed with rheumatoid arthritis. I was told to take methotrexate, which is a pretty serious drug; it's often used for cancer patients. I was concerned about the side effects, but the people at the center just kept telling me that everything was going to be ok, that lots of patients take this drug.

But they were also telling me I would have to take a flu shot because the drug would affect my immune system. This made me even more concerned. The nurse at the center just told me to think about it and decide what I wanted to do.

As luck would have it, at that time I found out about The Wellness Forum, attended a dinner and decided to become a member. I started attending classes and also joined the Physicians' Committee for Responsible Medicine to learn everything I could about diet. I eliminated dairy, reduced meat consumption to only a couple of times per week, and started eating lots of vegetables, rice, beans, and fruit.

Since joining The Wellness Forum, I haven't had any serious issues; once in a while I feel a little pain but nothing that keeps me from doing anything I want to do. I used to be really stiff when I'd been driving for a while or went to a movie. One time, a few weeks after I changed my diet I went to a movie and I just got right up and I walked right down the stairs and I just thought wow, I didn't even have trouble doing that. That was pretty amazing.

I no longer get headaches – I used to take Alleve two or three times per week, but I can't even remember the last time I had a headache. Although I wasn't planning to, I lost 30 pounds – I think that's just what happens when you start taking the bad things out of your diet. I had a few other health issues, such as low iron levels, which I was able to resolve with Dr. Pam's help.

I went back to the doctor a few times for blood tests and then decided not to go back. I remember asking my doctor if there was anything besides the drugs I could do for my condition, and he said there wasn't anything. He just encouraged me to take the drugs and told me everyone did and they were just fine. There was no sense in going back since I was not going to do anything he told me anyway.

I am so glad I decided not to take the drugs; I changed my diet, which not only improved the arthritis, but improved my weight and overall health too.

Aging Well!

It is exciting to talk about plant-based nutrition, particularly how the right diet can reverse conditions like heart disease, diabetes and even cancer. However, we do not want people to think that the diet is only for those who are sick; there are some great reasons for people currently in great health to adopt a well-structured plant-based diet. An obvious one is to maintain great health as you age - in other words, so that you can live until you die, rather than slowly degenerating over a long period of time.

There is a difference between your chronological age and your biological age. Your chronological age is the number of years you've been alive; plant-based nutrition and exercise cannot do anything to change that. Your biological age, on the other hand, is how fast you are wearing your body out and moving toward death. Nutrition, exercise and lifestyle choices have everything to do with your biological age.

We all see evidence of this difference in biological age in the people we know. Some people in their 60's look like they are 50 and have the energy of a 10-year-old, while others are in their 30's and have the appearance and energy levels of an elderly person.

Humans do not need to be overweight, or to develop common degenerative diseases; it is possible to remain healthy and vibrant and to do all of the things that you want to do as a senior!

Earl Bechtel's Story

I grew up on a farm in Ohio and we raised cattle, pigs and chickens. Every meal included meat and dairy. My mother was a great cook, so every meal also included dessert – home-based cookies, pies, and cakes.

I was athletic, which is one of the reasons why I didn't gain weight on this diet. I played football at Ohio State University for legendary coach Woody Hayes; this allowed my meat-based diet to continue through college and after.

My theory was that as long as I exercised and worked up a really good sweat, I could eat and drink whatever I wanted to. So, I'd start the day with 3-4 cups of coffee and some cigarettes. I'd play handball every day and right after, I'd eat a cheeseburger, French Fries and a milkshake, with more cigarettes as a chaser. Over the years, I put on some weight; my eating habits were the same but I was not exercising as much, and it showed.

I was fortunate to be invited to the very first Wellness 101 class taught in Dr. Pam Popper's home. I really was interested in learning about nutrition, and I started changing my diet. As I look back, I was lucky because other than my expanding waistline, I didn't have any major health issues. I look at my family now and realize that I could be like them. I have a brother who had carotid artery surgery and is dealing with kidney problems; a sister with health problems, and my brother was recently diagnosed with brain cancer. I, on the other hand, don't take any drugs at the age of 77 and I weigh only 5 pounds more than I did when I played college football!

About three years ago, I remarried and my new wife and I eat a pretty healthy plant-based diet with lots of rice, vegetables, and fruit. I learned how to make oil-free stir-fry and we make our own delicious pizzas without meat and cheese.

My quality of life is terrific. I work out at a fitness center close to my house a few times per week, travel, spend time with my grandkids, and I'm a professional foot reflexologist, which I love!

My diet is not perfect, but I really treasure the fact that Dr. Pam and The Wellness Forum are there to support me and keep me on track. I am particularly grateful for my life when I attend funeral services – lots of people in my age range are dying and I'm really living!

Most people don't believe I'm 77; I feel like I'm only 16, and I think this is the way humans are supposed to age.

Politics
And Health

Awakening Politically

Until a few years ago, I did not care about politics. I did not read newspapers or other publications in order to keep up with current events, and most of the time I didn't even bother to vote. I always knew who the President of the United States was, but most of the time didn't know who my state legislators or my Congressmen were. I justified my lack of interest with two observations that I frequently shared with others – first, it did not seem that much of what happened in politics had anything to do with me; and, I felt that one vote and one person could not make a difference in the outcome of anything anyway. I learned that I was wrong on both counts.

Lots of people feel like I did, and it seems like more and more people every year join the ranks of the politically apathetic. Here's the problem with this apathy. While many of us have been completely disinterested in politics, our elected officials have been busy passing laws that profoundly affect our lives, some in very negative ways. I learned that the more disinterested citizens like me become, the less elected officials feel like they have to answer to their constituents. If I don't show up to make my voice heard, politicians will listen to the people who do show up instead – lobbyists for special interest groups.

This chapter is about several things – it's about how I came to understand that not only is it in my best interest to get involved in government, but it's my responsibility as a citizen to do so. I cannot complain about what our government does if I am unwilling to become part of the solution by participating.

This section is also about how government, acting on behalf of and in conjunction with certain groups of medical professionals, pharmaceutical companies and other organizations with a financial interest in the health care industry, has been gradually restricting our health care choices, and the impact these restrictions can have on your life, your family's life, and your community.

Finally, it's about how you can help to change this situation by joining with a group of like-minded people who would like to end government interference in choices that should be ours to make.

247

It's time to take control of our government, our health and our future, but we cannot do it without engaging everyone in this effort. The largest special interest group in the U.S. consists of people who want to make their own decisions about health – if all of us join together and pool our resources, we'll be able to outspend the pharmaceutical companies, the practice groups, insurance companies and many others who work hard to preserve their monopoly. And, we'll be able to convince politicians that their ability to be re-elected depends, in part, on their willingness to represent the voters who want reform in this area.

A Visit From the State

The story of my experience with state government is important because it was the catalyst for what has become an important part of my life's work – changing laws that restrict consumer choice. Sharing it is also important because what happened to me can happen to anyone!

I never expected to be a target of a state investigation, and I was so naïve that when I occasionally heard about people who were investigated by the government, I assumed that those people had done something terribly wrong. I believed that government needed a reason to intrude on our lives. Thus, I was very shocked when the State of Ohio began an investigation of me and The Wellness Forum in 1997.

As I mentioned earlier in this book, when I decided to pursue education in the nutrition field, I looked into becoming a dietitian and determined that this educational pathway was not for me. I was not interested in working in an institutional food service operation, disagreed with the philosophy of dietetics in general, and was opposed to the cozy financial relationship that the American Dietetic Association had with food manufacturers and agricultural groups. I decided to pursue an alternative education, which was less than ideal, but closer to my philosophy. It never occurred to me that talking to people about nutrition as a non-dietitian could be illegal.

I was first contacted by the Ohio State Board of Dietetics in April, 1997. According to the letter I received, the Board had received an inquiry about our "weight control program." The Wellness Forum did not at that time offer a "weight control program," and I was unaware that State agencies investigate businesses based on "inquiries." Nonetheless, in the spirit of cooperation, I submitted answers to the questions included in the letter from the Board and received a letter from the Board some months later indicating that The Wellness Forum was in compliance with the law. I thought that the matter was closed.

The next time I heard from the Board was via a telephone call from the Board's investigator, Beth Shaffer, in mid-1998. Ms. Shaffer was investigating a company called "Fitness Resources," a private gym in Columbus. According to Ms. Shaffer, someone had picked up one of our brochures at Fitness Resources and forwarded it to Ms. Shaffer. She had several questions about the services we offered, as well as questions about the activities of Fitness Resources. During this conversation, which lasted for about 40 minutes, Ms. Shaffer also questioned me about Fitness Resources' Board of Advisors and several other people in the health care field and their activities. I answered the questions to the best of my knowledge, but was unable to provide any substantial information. Although I knew the owner of Fitness Resources, it was not my business. Again, at this time I thought cooperation was the best approach.

In February, 1999, Ms. Shaffer again contacted me, stating that she had several questions about The Wellness Forum and wanted to meet with me personally. Ms. Shaffer informed me that a complaint had been filed against The Wellness Forum concerning a lecture called "Raw Food and Weight Loss." As a result of this complaint, she wanted to see the lecture notes from that presentation.

Again, I tried to be cooperative, thinking that this was the best way to handle the situation, so I agreed to meet her. The meeting took place on February 23 and I took notes both during and after the meeting. When asked who filed the complaint, or the nature of the complaint, Ms. Shaffer informed me that she did not have to provide me with that information. I did provide her with the notes from the lecture, but Ms. Shaffer continued to ask questions about other events on our calendar, and the speakers and their credentials. I knew this was not going to end well when Ms. Shaffer informed me during this meeting that showing the movie *Diet for a New America* could be considered the unlicensed practice of dietetics (a misdemeanor crime in Ohio) because watching it might make someone change their dietary habits.

At one time, she told me that she was very concerned because people who are not dietitians often use titles like "nutritionist" to describe themselves and their activities. In response to this, I gave Ms. Shaffer a copy of a cookbook I had authored in which I stated clearly in the Forward that I was not a nutritionist or dietitian. I thought that this cookbook might give her some assurance that I did not misrepresent my credentials to the public.

Ms. Shaffer became rude and confrontational during this meeting. She told me to inform one of the speakers listed on our calendar that she should not use the title "Dr." because people might confuse her with a "real doctor." (This practitioner was a naturopathic physician with two Ph.D.'s). She also asked if I knew anything about my landlord, a chiropractor, because she had heard that he was giving out nutritional advice and she might start an investigation of him. (Interesting, since nutrition is within the scope of practice for chiropractors in Ohio).

I asked Ms. Shaffer about my rights to free speech under the First Amendment, as it pertains to public lectures and I was informed that "there are no First Amendment Rights in the State of Ohio when it comes to discussions about food and nutrition."

At one time during our encounter, I suggested to Ms. Shaffer that I would prefer not to have such a confrontational interchange with her, to which she replied, "I am not here to be your friend. You can think of me like the police. I am an enforcer for the State of Ohio." By this time I was getting angry and informed Ms. Shaffer that I wasn't planning to ask her to play golf with me, but was simply wondering if we could be civil. After a little more hostile exchange, she left.

Based on the confrontational and hostile tone of this meeting, I retained a Registered Dietitian, Denise Londergan, to supervise the activities at The Wellness Forum and to certify to the Board, if there were further inquiries, that we were not engaged in the practice of dietetics. I am deeply indebted to Denise and to many other forward-thinking health care professionals for being our friends and allies during this period of time, and for helping us in our quest to change the laws in response to incidents like these.

A few months later, in June, I received a certified letter, signed by the Executive Director of the Ohio Board of Dietetics, Kay Mavko, requesting the following:

- The names and credentials of the individuals presenting workshops called "Cooking Lite" and "Fiber: The Neglected Nutrient," as well as information (again) pertaining to the lecture "Raw Food and Weight Loss."
- The names of instructors, as well as class outlines for everything on our calendar, which included such events as exercise workshops, stress workshops and yoga, which were clearly outside of the jurisdiction of the Board.
- The names of people who had received "nutrition services," even though I had repeatedly told the Board and demonstrated to them that we did not provide "nutrition services" at that time.

In the letter, Ms. Mavko referred to a cookbook and an enzyme book used in our "weight control program." The Board had been told repeatedly that The Wellness Forum did not offer a program of weight control. Ms. Shaffer was told that the enzyme book was provided by the manufacturer of a food product we sold, and the cookbook was provided simply as a courtesy to her because the Forward provided written evidence that I was not misrepresenting my credentials. Ms. Shaffer evidently either did not tell Ms. Mavko about our meeting or misrepresented what I said.

On June 10, I faxed a letter to Kay Mavko responding to her inquiry. Again, I stated that The Wellness Forum did not offer a program of weight control and that enzyme book provided to Ms. Shaffer was provided to me by a manufacturer, which is covered by an exemption in the law; and that the cookbook had been given to Ms. Shaffer only for her to see the Forward, which stated in writing that I was not a dietitian. I explained that I had taught the "Cooking Lite" class and that there were no lecture notes, as I was comfortable doing cooking demonstrations without notes since I write cookbooks. I also informed Ms. Mavko that I had hired a dietitian to supervise our activities and to assure the Board that we were not engaging in the practice of dietetics.

Within a few days, Ms. Shaffer called Denise Londergan. She was rude and confrontational, which seemed to be her general style of communication. When Ms. Londergan said that she was suffering from allergies and found it difficult to talk, Ms. Shaffer responded that she doubted it was allergies, but rather nerves due to the nature of the Ohio Board of Dietetics inquiry. At one point Ms. Londergan informed Ms. Shaffer that she felt that Ms. Shaffer was uninterested in her responses to questions unless those responses were the ones Ms. Shaffer was seeking. Ms. Londergan contacted me immediately at the conclusion of the telephone call with Ms. Shaffer, and expressed concern about the intentions of the Board.

Later, on that same day, Ms. Shaffer left a message on my voice mail informing me that the Board of Dietetics was launching a formal investigation of The Wellness Forum and that she expected to hear from me immediately on this matter. Since all attempts at cooperation on my part had failed, I retained a lawyer to represent me.

My attorney, C. Michael Piacentino, met with Ms. Mavko and Ms. Shaffer and during this meeting, they informed him that they were investigating both me and The Wellness Forum and failure to respond to their requests would result in subpoenas and other strong actions by the Board. The areas of inquiry were centered around the public lectures: "Raw Food and Weight Loss," "Cooking Lite" and "Fiber: The Neglected Nutrient." During this meeting the Board finally agreed to stop asking about "Raw Food and Weight Loss" since they had been told on numerous occasions about the details of this lecture. Mr. Piacentino told me after the meeting that he also was concerned about the Board's intentions. It appeared to him that they had made up their mind to pursue me, and that the presentation of evidence that we had done nothing wrong would not likely dissuade them.

The regulations governing the dietetics laws showed that we were on very solid ground in presenting the public lectures and classes about which the Board was inquiring. Under "Definitions," the practice of dietetics in the Ohio Revised Code is defined as follows:

> (A) Nutritional assessment means the integrative evaluation of nutritionally relevant data to develop an **individualized care plan**.
> (B) Nutritional counseling means the advising of individuals or groups regarding nutritional intake based on **individual** needs.
> (C) Nutrition education means a planned program based on learning objectives with expected outcomes designed to modify nutrition-related behaviors.   (emphasis mine)

I and no one else I have consulted can understand how a public lecture on fiber or a cooking class can possibly be interpreted to mean the practice of dietetics based on these criteria.

My attorney responded to the Board via certified letter in September 1999. The letter reviewed the fact that The Wellness Forum was not engaged in the practice of dietetics based on the definitions in the Ohio Revised Code because the lectures did not include any elements of nutritional assessment, counseling, or education based on individual needs.

For several months, we did not hear from the Board. On May 19, 2000, Ms. Shaffer contacted me at my home. She asked me for a current copy of the calendar of events for The Wellness Forum. This time she told me that the reason more information was needed was that the Board of Dietetics had filed a complaint against The Wellness Forum with the Ohio Consumer Protection Agency, and that this agency had found our company to be in violation of some statute. I reminded her that I had a lawyer and that she should contact him.

The following week, Ms. Mavko called Mr. Piacentino to ask for a copy of the calendar, again citing the Ohio Consumer Protection Agency's ruling as the reason for the request. Mr. Piacentino asked her to provide a copy of the Ohio Consumer Protection Agency's findings, since we could not possibly comply with a ruling we knew nothing about, and to put her request for information in writing.

Two days later, Ms. Shaffer called Mr. Piacentino and demanded a copy of the calendar. His response was the same. By this time, this investigation was starting to cost me a lot of money. Every time the board contacted me and a response was required, I incurred a bill from my lawyer. This is one of the reasons it's hard for citizens to stand up to the government. Government officials have the unlimited resources of the state at their disposal – they don't have to worry about funding their investigations and expenses. Citizens like you and I have to pay for our own legal fees and expenses. This, I learned, is why many people either settle by agreeing to anything asked of them, or simply go out of business when faced with similar circumstances. I refused to do either – I was determined to see this incident through to the end regardless of the consequences financially or otherwise.

On June 1, 2000, the Board sent Mr. Piacentino a letter requesting the name of each workshop presented since January, 1999, the name of the presenter and his or her credentials, along with an outline of each program, and any advertisements used to promote these lectures.

This information was virtually impossible to provide since many of the speakers were guest speakers rather than associates of The Wellness Forum, and we did not keep their bios and lecture notes on file (this was before computers kept track of everything – our calendars were produced on typewriters at that time!). In addition, many of the workshops were related to topics like stress and exercise that had nothing to do with food, and therefore were outside the Board's jurisdiction.

Again, Mr. Piacentino asked for the ruling from the Ohio Consumer Protection Agency, and again Ms. Mavko refused to deliver it.

At this time, a close friend, Linda Reidelbach, was running for election to the Ohio House of Representatives. She had been a political activist for a while, so I contacted her and sent her my file, and the files of others who had come forward who had similar experiences with this same Board. She reviewed the files, agreed that there seemed to be something amiss, and contacted then-State Representative Pat Tiberi. Rep. Tiberi had been involved in an investigation of the Ohio State Dental Board for over-zealous regulatory tactics against dentists and she thought he would be interested in my case. He read the files and also concluded that there was indeed a problem and agreed to conduct a meeting in his office in an attempt to mediate the situation. The Board of Dietetics insisted that the meeting be only with me and not include the other people who had grievances with the Board. I insisted that my lawyer attend the meeting, however.

It took several weeks for the meeting to take place, and by that time, Mr. Tiberi had decided to run for national office and was quite involved with his campaign. He delegated the meeting to a new staff assistant, Beth O'Boyle.

On August 29, Mr. Piacentino and I met with Ms. Mavko and Sally DeBolt from the Ohio Attorney General's Office, with Beth O'Boyle presiding. The meeting was generally unproductive. The discussion centered around legal and constitutional issues with which Beth had little familiarity. She made every effort to not take sides, or to do anything at all.

After 90 acrimonious minutes, we agreed that the Board would pare down its request to a reasonable size and would provide us with the ruling from The Ohio Consumer Protection Agency.

Within one week, Mr. Piacentino's office received a request from Ms. Mavko that was slightly more cumbersome than the original one. Although the request included a copy of the minutes describing the Board's decision to file a complaint with the Ohio Consumer Protection Agency, it did not include the ruling, claiming it to be "work product."

Mr. Piacentino responded to Ms. Mavko's letter, again requesting the ruling from the Ohio Consumer Protection Agency.

Ms. Mavko responded by stating that we had misunderstood the agreement in Representative Tiberi's office and refused to provide the complaint or the ruling from the Ohio Consumer Protection Agency.

A subpoena was issued immediately for the information the Board was seeking, but I was traveling at the time and it was not successfully served.

In the meantime, I contacted State Representative Jim Hughes. Rep. Hughes had been contacted by constituents in his district who were experiencing or had experienced similar problems with the Ohio Board of Dietetics. Representative Hughes wrote Ms. Mavko a letter stating that he had reviewed my file and a few others' files and had some serious concerns about the activities of the Board. He asked that all activity stop until he could investigate and sort it out. Ms. Mavko replied that the subpoena had already been issued and that she could do nothing about it.

The original subpoena expired. Ms. Shaffer again called me at home to inform me that another subpoena had been issued and delivered to my housekeeper. I again told Ms. Shaffer to stop calling me directly and to please talk to my attorney.

Ms. Shaffer then called Mr. Piacentino and asked him if he would accept the subpoena on my behalf. He replied that he would not.

Following these conversations, Mr. Hughes called Ms. Mavko and informed her that since the subpoenas had all expired, there was no reason not to stop the investigation pending his own investigation. Ms. Mavko refused to cooperate and stated that the Board intended to continue to pursue me.

The Board was successful in serving me with a subpoena in early December. At this time, Mr. Piacentino recommended that I retain another attorney who was more experienced in this arena, which caused my legal bills started to escalate dramatically. His recommendation for additional counsel was made, in part, because the minutes for the Board's November meeting stated, "The Board determined that it should exercise all authority within its power to enforce the issuance and compliance with the subpoena ordered." Legally, this meant that the Board could bring me to court on a show-cause order, where failure to produce the requested material would result in imprisonment for contempt. In these cases, the term of imprisonment is either until the material is turned over, or a judge decides that no length of time in jail will compel the defendant to produce the material. Mr. Piacentino was justifiably concerned about the chance that I might have to spend some time in jail.

My primary objection to providing the Board with what they requested was that one of the items they asked for was a list of people who had spoken at our center. I had no intention of providing this aggressive agency with names and addresses of other people so they could begin investigations of them like the one I had been enduring for the past three years. I would rot in jail before I would subject others to this treatment. I later found out that I was right about this. Employees of the Board admitted during testimony in front of a legislative committee that they often started "secondary investigations" of people who were identified while investigating another target.

By this time, we were able to access the minutes of the November 2000 Board meeting in which a Cease and Desist Order that they had voted to issue against me on December 3, 1999 was referenced. I had not, as of this time, received such an order. This was an interesting revelation; if the Board had enough information to issue a Cease and Desist order in December, 1999, why were they continuing to investigate me throughout the following year? Was this pure harassment? Or, had they decided to issue a Cease and Desist order prior to having any information (in other words, determining guilt in advance). Neither scenario places the Board's intentions in a good light.

The new member of my legal team, David Frank, explained to me that there was a chance that refusing to turn over the requested information would result in jail time, and we perceived the threat to be serious enough to begin figuring out how the company would operate without me, who would take care of my cat, pay college tuition for my daughter, etc. My parents offered to provide financial assistance if necessary. I really started to believe that I was headed for incarceration. This was a really stressful time in my life.

My attorney responded to the Board's subpoena, basically informing them that we would not be providing the information requested.

By this time, Linda Reidelbach had been elected to office, and mentioned my situation to then-Governor Taft at the Governor's Holiday Party. I had spoken to Governor Taft about my case at a fundraiser earlier that year, and he remembered the conversation. He was flabbergasted that the case had progressed to the point that incarceration was a possibility. He suggested that she call Bill Klatt, his legal counsel.

Mr. Klatt contacted me and, although very careful not to take sides, expressed some concern about the Board's interpretation of the law, and whether or not a judge would uphold that interpretation. He subsequently communicated this to the Board, as well as the fact that both Representatives Reidelbach and Hughes were concerned about the Board's activities.

Mr. Klatt was successful in getting the Board to provide us with the ruling from the Consumer Protection Section of the Ohio Attorney General's Office. (We discovered at this time that there was no such agency as the Ohio Consumer Protection Agency) I also subsequently discovered that Ms. Shaffer and employees of the Board had used this fictitious agency to threaten others who were targets of investigations as well. The complaint was made to the Attorney General's office by the Board, not by a consumer, and the information in the complaint was false. The complaint alleged that we were holding lectures with the intent of selling food without disclosing that intent in our promotional materials. We have never claimed that the purpose of our lectures was to sell food. We claimed that our lectures were covered under the right to free speech. In other words, the Board made a complaint based on false information and used the response to its false complaint to justify another two years of investigation of our activities.

During the month of January, 2001, the Board continued to harass me and other associates of The Wellness Forum. Ms. Shaffer contacted the owner of The Wellness Forum in Grand Rapids, Michigan posing as a prospective client. She attempted to get in touch with a dietitian who worked with that center through the American Dietetic Association. To my knowledge, the Ohio Board of Dietetics has no jurisdiction in Michigan.

Ms. Shaffer contacted Bowling Green State University, where a nurse practitioner associated with The Wellness Forum, Dr. Sue Ryno, was teaching workshops on nutrition. Ms. Shaffer was following up on a call she received from a Registered Dietitian who was upset that she was not asked to teach the nutrition classes at BGSU.
The Board insists that it only follows up on complaints. I do not understand how a dietitian upset about a lost business opportunity constitutes a "complaint."

Dr. Ryno's scope of practice, and indeed her agreement with her collaborating physician, which is filed with the state, includes nutrition education. Bowling Green is an accredited institution, and is covered under an exemption in the Ohio Revised Code Section 4759.10 (D):
> "Persons employed by a non-profit agency approved by the board or by a federal, state, municipal or county government, or by any other political subdivision, elementary or secondary school, or an institution of higher education approved by the board or by a regional agency recognized by the council on postsecondary accreditation..."

Did Ms. Shaffer not know that Bowling Green was an accredited institution? Or was she unsure that Dr. Ryno was a nurse practitioner? It seems that the objective of this inquiry was simply to harass and interfere with our business relationships.

Ms. Shaffer also contacted the Director of Nursing Education at Northwest Community College, through which The Wellness Forum offered Continuing Education Programs for nurses, inferring to the Director of Nursing that The Wellness Forum and I should not be allowed to provide nursing CE's. Northwestern Community College is an accredited non-profit educational institution; its activities are not under the jurisdiction of the Ohio Board of Dietetics. The Board also has no jurisdiction over the Ohio Board of Nursing, its providers and approvers. Non-dietitians routinely offer courses related to nutrition and many other topics both in the classroom and in a home-study format for nursing CE's, so the arrangement was not atypical. Again, the purpose of the inquiry seemed to be simply harassment.

We spent a lot of time and effort during this period just responding to people and institutions who were contacted by Ms. Shaffer. Thankfully, we did not lose on client, affiliation, or relationship as a result of this harassment. If the goal of the Ohio Board of Dietetics was to put us out of business, the agency must have been quite frustrated by now. I'll be forever thankful for those who stuck by us during this time.

Concerned about the communication from Bill Klatt about the Board's activities, Ms. Mavko and Ms Shaffer met with both Representatives Reidelbach and Hughes prior to the January 2001, meeting of the Ohio Board of Dietetics. According to both of these Representatives, Ms. Mavko and Ms. Shaffer appeared to be trying to assess how upset these politicians were, and the political implications of taking action against me.

Although we'll never know the specifics of the discussion at the Board meeting regarding the disposition of my case, the minutes show that after spending two years of trying to get me to produce names and addresses, lecture notes, and other information, the Board abandoned that effort and decided to finally issue a cease and desist order against me and The Wellness Forum. Many of the activities listed in the cease and desist are exempt under Ohio statute or are covered by my rights to free speech. My attorneys replied to the Board with the same information we've been providing for years:

- The Wellness Forum and I were not engaged in the practice of dietetics as defined by Ohio law.
- Many of our activities are covered by our rights to free speech as guaranteed by the First Amendment to the United States Constitution and Article I, section 11 of the Ohio Constitution.

Subsequent to the cease and desist order, I received still another letter from the Board stating that I could no longer use my earned credentials, which included Ph.D.

The Board's problem with my use of the earned credential, "Ph.D.," is their allegation that the school that granted my degrees is not accredited by the American Dietetic Association. I specifically sought an education *not* sanctioned by the American Dietetic Association, since I do not agree with much of the information that is provide by this organization and its licensees, and I dislike the financial relationship the ADA has with food producers.

It seemed that finally this debacle had come to an end, and we simply continued to do what we had been doing since the business started in my family room several years ago. Nothing changed, including the use of my earned credentials on my business card. But this ordeal was extraordinarily expensive, costing tens of thousands of dollars. In addition to the out-of-pocket expenses, I spent entire work-weeks dealing with the Board and its harassment. The time spent definitely affected revenues at the company. The fear associated with potentially spending some time in jail for not complying with the subpoena was immeasurable, not only for me, but for my family.

The Board's harassment did not result in the loss of any business relationships, but did result in embarrassment and stress, as we had to constantly explain the situation to people who were being contacted by the Board's investigator. Most people were very understanding and, in fact, agreed after their contacts with Ms. Shaffer that the Board's activities were out of line..
I did not breathe a sigh of relief, however. I knew that sooner or later this board would be back if I did not do something proactive to change the laws under which they were able to pursue me the way that they did. And thus my career as a political activist began.

Although my interest began with a desire to change the dietetics laws in Ohio, I soon discovered that the laws governing the practice of other occupations were just as restrictive, and that Ohio was not the only state in which these types of problems existed.

There are so many practitioners who have been investigated by so many state boards in so many states that an entire book could be written just to tell their stories. I've chosen to include just one more in order to make the point that *many* state licensure boards misbehave; not just the Ohio Board of Dietetics.

Dan Nuzum's Story

Dan Nuzum was a naturopath in Toledo, Ohio who faced 5th degree felony charges as a result of an investigation by the Ohio Chiropractic Board.

Dan studied at the North American College of Naproprathic Medicine in Arkansas and graduated in 1997. He then enrolled in the Southern College of Naturopathic Medicine in Mexico, where he spent 2 years and received a Naturopathic Medical Degree.

In 2000, Dan moved to Ohio to work with Dr. Robert McKinney at Central States College of Health Sciences, and joined the teaching staff at the school.

Dr. Nuzum opened his office in Toledo, Ohio in January 2003. In April 2004 the Ohio Chiropractic Board opened an investigation of Dr. Nuzum's practice. An undercover police officer visited the office with a hidden camera and obtained footage of Dan performing mechanotherapy on a patient.

On November 9, investigators from the chiropractic and medical boards, along with a police officer and SWAT team officers in full gear raided his office. They interrogated 8 patients, an office assistant and nurses. They threatened to arrest anyone that did not provide a full name and social security number. Dan was arrested, handcuffed, and taken to jail, where he spent the night and the next day incarcerated with a rapist and convicted murderer. He had no prior criminal record. He was eventually released on his own recognizance.

Police officers who know Dan told him that they have never seen a person arrested in this manner for a 5th degree felony. They said that people are usually given an opportunity to turn themselves in. Surprise arrest and immediate incarceration is reserved for those who have a criminal record, are a threat to public safety, or a flight risk.

Dan believes it was a chiropractor who suggested that the Board look into his activities, rather than a complaint from a bona fide patient. This is most likely true. State Representative Linda Reidelbach reviewed over 100 cases investigated by The Ohio Board of Dietetics, and found that there were no *consumer* complaints; the complaints came from other licensed dietitians and employees of the board, who regularly spent time looking through the phone book, gathering information from flyers posted in health food stores, and looking for signs on buildings in order to dig up targets for investigation.

On December 15, 2005, Dr. Nuzum's case went to trial. He was found not guilty by the Court.

Unfortunately, and this is so often the case, Dr. Nuzum won his case, but at tremendous cost. The police confiscated his computers and equipment, which essentially closed his practice the day he was raided, and prevented him from earning a living. His legal fees totaled tens of thousands of dollars. The investigation was widely covered by the media, effectively ruining his name in the Toledo area. And, his patients were deprived of their health care practitioner during this period of time.

Few people have the funds or the intestinal fortitude to endure the stress, threat of criminal prosecution, loss of livelihood and other circumstances associated with heavy-handed government intervention. This is why it is imperative that we change the laws that allow this activity.

Understanding Licensure

Economist Milton Friedman published an essay over 40 years ago called *Capitalism and Freedom* in which he stated "The pressure on the legislature to license an occupation rarely comes from the members of the public who have been mulcted. On the contrary, the pressure invariably comes from members of the occupation itself."

This is true. Professionals ranging from frog farmers to medical doctors have been seeking licensure, which is regulated at the state level, for decades. The number of licensed professions has grown and continues to grow. And in almost every case, legislation to license a group is proposed by the professional group itself.

Legislators are told that licensure is necessary to protect the public. According to practice groups, requiring certain educational pathways, a clear scope of practice, and supervision by state employees who have the power to revoke licensure if a practitioner misbehaves, protects the public from harm.

This, however, is not the most important reason that health care professionals seek licensure. Licensure laws are often strategies for restricting competition.

The reality is that few people are hurt by non-licensed practitioners. Yet professional groups have used scare tactics for decades to convince legislators that not only should their group be licensed, but that everyone who is not a member of their group should be prevented from practicing.

At one time, medical doctors were licensed to practice medicine, and osteopaths were not. Medical doctors spent enormous amounts of time and money convincing state legislators and the public that osteopaths were dangerous and a threat to public safety.

Eventually, osteopaths gained licensure and they quickly joined with the medical doctors to make sure that everyone knew that chiropractors were threats to public safety. In fact, the American Chiropractic Association filed a lawsuit alleging restraint of trade, among other counts, against the American Medical Association (AMA) and other defendants. In 1987, the courts ruled in their favor, with an opinion stating, "...In the early 1960's, the AMA decided to contain and eliminate chiropractic as a profession. In 1963, the AMA Committee on Quackery was formed. The committee worked aggressively, both overtly and covertly to eliminate chiropractic."[245]

Partly as a result of this court decision, chiropractors have gained licensure and they have joined other licensed occupations in trying to keep new groups of professionals like naturopaths from being able to legally practice. It's time for this behavior to stop!

During the 12 years I've been working on legislative reform in Ohio that would allow non-licensed practitioners such as non-dietitians, naturopaths, herbalists, and various body workers to practice, the 11 boards governing the licensure of health care professionals have been unable to produce one Ohioan who has been hurt by a non-licensed practitioner. They certainly have an incentive to produce a person who has been harmed, and I'm in possession of a communication from one of these boards asking its licensees to dig up a harmed person because it would help to kill our legislation. Yet, not one person, so far, has come forward claiming to have been hurt. If no one is being harmed, why are licensed practitioners so vehement in opposing access to these practitioners?

Since licensure laws are proposed by practice groups, they are often very broadly written, granting broad rule-writing authority to the licensure board once it is formed. The rule-writing process outlines details for the enforcement of the law, and as long as they don't stray too far from the statutes, boards can write very restrictive rules.

Until recently, most licensure laws were passed without members of the public or other groups of health care practitioners even knowing about them. Little, if any, attention was paid to the writing of the rules and regulations. Over time, members of the various boards in many states wrote and imposed increasingly strong and limiting rules and regulations that made it easier and easier to investigate and prosecute professionals who were not members of the protected groups.

This has started to change. The availability of information via the internet, and increased ease of communications among both citizens and practitioner groups has resulted in the defeat of many proposed licensure laws, modification of some laws that have passed, and more attention paid to the rule-writing process in order to stop predatory behavior.

Dietitian Licensure

Almost all states license dietitians. The dietetics lobby is a powerful and persistent one, and in spite of being unable to prove that lack of regulation in the nutrition business presents a threat to public health, efforts to license dietitians have been successful.

The problem with dietitian licensure laws is not the licensure of dietitians, per se, but rather the additional provisions that are included in most laws that have prevented people who have training that is different and sometimes even better than dietitians, from dispensing nutrition advice. These provisions include title protection, in which dietitians claim ownership of any designation that might indicate that an individual has expertise in the area of nutrition. No one objects to dietitians being the only ones able to use the terms "Registered Dietitian" or "Licensed Dietitian." But in many states, including Ohio, dietitians claim ownership of all other related names as well.

For example, Ohio Revised Code Section 47759.02 (B) (2) states:
"No person except for a person licensed under Chapters 4701. to 4755. of the Revised Code, when acting within the scope of their practice, shall use any other title, designation, words, letters, abbreviation, or insignia, or other combination of any title, designation, words, letters, abbreviation, or insignia tending to indicate that the person is practicing dietetics."

The Board has used this statute as a basis for investigating people who use titles such as "Certified Nutritionist," "Certified Clinical Nutritionist" and other earned titles, claiming that these titles lead people to believe that an individual is practicing dietetics.

I know several people who have been investigated by the Ohio Board of Dietetics for using titles such as "nutritionist," and the use of my own credentials was an issue in the Board's investigation and actions against me.

Citizens Can Make a Difference!

In 2001, several people who had been investigated by the Ohio Board of Dietetics worked on a bill that would end the dietitians' monopoly over nutrition practices in Ohio. These people included Claudia David, a well-known health food store owner and political activist from Toledo, Patty Shipley, me, and many others who testified in front of committees, wrote letters and met with legislators.

Although the bill did not pass, so much pressure was applied by legislators in response to testimony and letters from the public, that the Ohio Board of Dietetics was forced to amend its rules to allow for "non-medical nutrition education" to be offered by non-dietitians.

"Non-medical nutrition education" included:
  (1) Principles of good nutrition and food preparation
  (2) Food to be included in the normal daily diet
  (3) The essential nutrients needed by the body
  (4) Recommended amounts of essential nutrients
  (5) The actions of nutrients on the body
  (6) The effects of excesses or deficiencies of nutrients; or
  (7) Food or supplements that are good sources of essential nutrients

This provision legalized much of the activity that had been the subject of investigations by the board, but the law still prevents non-dietitians from using their earned credentials, and from counseling clients about personal health issues. Ohio still needs legislative reform.

Coco Newton is a forward-thinking and enlightened Registered Dietitian in Michigan who found out that a dietetics bill much like Ohio's was flying through the Michigan State legislature. Determined to prevent the Michigan legislature from putting non-dietitian nutrition professionals out of business, she hurriedly prepared testimony for the Senate committee considering the bill, consulted with a lawyer, and was successful in producing a sub-bill that included several provisions protecting many types of nutrition practitioners and the rights of Michigan residents to choose their nutrition professionals. This bill was the one that became law.

For example, one section of the bill states "The Department, in consultation with the Board, shall not promulgate rules under this section that diminish competition or exceed the minimum level of regulation necessary to protect the public." This is the type of language that can prevent the Board from developing

Administrative Rules that prohibit competition, as has been done in so many other states.

In addition to working on the language in the bill, Coco was appointed to serve as a member of the Michigan Board of Dietetics, along with another enlightened dietitian, Mohey Mowafy, Ph.D., R.D., CNS, CEDS. These two individuals are diligently working to make sure that Michigan's dietetics law is interpreted according to the intent of the legislation, which was to regulate dietetic practice, not to eliminate competition.

These are just two examples of what can happen when citizens decide to make their voices heard.

Anthropologist Margaret Mead once said, "Never doubt that a small group of thoughtful, committed citizens can change the world. Indeed, it is the only thing that ever has."

Naturopathic Licensure

There is a great deal of confusion and disagreement about licensure for naturopaths. This confusion stems from a basic misunderstanding about the difference between the practice of **naturopathy** and the practice of **naturopathic medicine**.

The best definition of naturopathy I have seen appeared on the website for the Coalition for Natural Health:

"Naturopathy: a distinct system of non-invasive healthcare and health assessment in which neither surgery nor drugs are used, dependence being placed only on education, counseling, naturopathic modalities and natural substances, including without limitation, the use of foods, food extracts, vitamins, minerals, enzymes, digestive aids, botanical substances, topical natural substances, homeopathic preparations, air, water, heat, cold, sound, light, the physical modalities of magnetic therapy, naturopathic non-manipulative bodywork and exercise to help stimulate and maintain the individual's intrinsic self-healing processes."

In other words, naturopaths focus on educating clients about the use of natural substances to promote health. A classically trained naturopath does not diagnose disease, does not serve as a primary care physician, does not prescribe drugs, and does not instruct individuals to discontinue their relationship with or to stop following the advice of their physicians.

Naturopathic physicians, on the other hand, are trained to practice naturopathic medicine. They attend a four-year residential program, which is currently offered by four accredited schools in the U.S. They can diagnose and treat disease, prescribe drugs, perform surgery, deliver babies, and are trained to be primary care physicians.

Naturopathic physicians are licensed in some states, and are seeking licensure in many others. I and most others support licensure for these doctors.

The problem is that the American Association of Naturopathic Physicians (AANP) has proposed legislation that not only licenses graduates of these four-year schools, but prevents classically trained naturopaths from practicing. The bills also include title protection, tying up all terms associated with "naturopathy" and reserving them only for use by the graduates of these four-year schools.

This is reminiscent of the turf-protecting, onerous dietetics licensure laws that were passed in many states, and that almost everyone (except most dietitians) now agrees were a terrible idea. Enormous amounts of time and resources have been spent on legal defense, and trying to reform these laws in Ohio and in other states.

One of the wonderful things about the information age is that lots of people are now aware of the AANP and its legislative activities, and have worked together to block its legislation. Several groups lobbied successfully in Colorado to defeat AANP's licensure bill in 2008. Opposition to a similar bill in Missouri in 2006 resulted in the legislature's decision to table the issue of naturopathic licensure indefinitely. The Missouri Senate Interim Committee on Naturopathic Medicine included this statement in its final report, "The committee feels that it has come to an understanding of the definition and components of naturopathy and naturopathic medicine. However, it remains unclear to the committee who is a naturopath and what makes one a naturopath. This is a fundamental and necessary question that the committee was unable to determine. The committee, at this time, recommends against licensure of Naturopathic physicians in the state of Missouri."

The answer, in my opinion, is to allow classically trained naturopaths to practice under exemption legislation (covered next), and to license naturopathic physicians to practice with a scope of practice that reflects their training. Instead of fighting with one another, the two groups should be working together to ensure freedom for everyone to practice responsibly.

Exemption Bills

In most states, a few groups of health care professionals are licensed. These include physicians, nurses, dentists, occupational and physical therapists, psychologists, and dietitians. There are many health care occupations that are not licensed, including herbalists, Certified Nutritionists, nutrition professionals with alternative training, classically trained naturopaths, energy healers, and body workers such as rolfers, shiatsu massage therapists, polarity practitioners, and many more.

In most states the offering of these modalities is considered the unlicensed practice of some occupation, and in some states is a criminal offense. State licensure boards do not need a consumer complaint or any evidence of harm in order to begin an investigation of a non-licensed practitioner – they simply need to know that the practitioner is in business. As you learned earlier, the boards often encourage their licensees to turn in practitioners, and some are all too happy to cooperate. This causes many practitioners to operate underground since they fear prosecution, which can make it difficult for consumers to find practitioners when they need them.

Although it may seem on the surface that licensing all of these practitioners would solve the problem, there are many obstacles to licensing each of these groups:
  • It is expensive to get licensure laws passed, since it is almost impossible to do so without an organized effort

and a lobbyist. Although there may be tens of thousands of non-licensed practitioners in each state engaged in some form of practice, there are usually not enough engaged in each occupation, for example foot reflexologists, to fund such an effort for each practice group.

- Licensed occupations are expected to fund their regulatory offices through licensure fees. Many of these practice groups are not large enough to fund such an office through licensure fees.

- Some people have suggested the formation of a single board to regulate all non-licensed practitioners. This is not practical, however. The concept of licensure is to standardize educational requirements, and to develop a specific scope of practice. This would be almost impossible to do effectively for dozens of different types of practitioners. People learn herbal medicine through distance learning courses, certification programs, and apprenticeship, for example. Which method of training would be the accepted one? List all three as acceptable and surely a new one will surface that had not been previously considered. Think about the difficulty of a board doing this for dozens of different types of practices, many of which the board members know little or nothing about.

The State of Minnesota passed legislation in 2000 which legalized these practices through a process of exemption, rather than through licensure. Exemption bills are usually called Health Freedom Bills or Consumer Health Freedom Bills. The health freedom movement will forever be indebted to Minnesota attorney Diane Miller, who worked tirelessly to get the Minnesota bill passed, which paved the way for similar legislation in a few other states. I am hopeful that eventually all states will pass these laws.

Exemption laws allow all non-licensed practitioners to practice, provided they meet two criteria:
- They must give each client a disclosure document that informs the consumer that the practitioner is not licensed by the state, describes the services offered, how fees are charged, and other pertinent information.

271

- The practitioners must agree to not engage in a list of prohibited activities that are to be performed by licensed practitioners only. In other words, what differentiates non-licensed from licensed professionals is their *scope of practice.*

Although this varies from state to state, the following list is a typical prohibited activity list:
- The performance of surgery or any other procedure that punctures the skin
- The performance of any adjustment of the joints or spine
- The recommendation of any procedure that involves ionizing radiation
- Diagnosis of a disease
- Diagnosis or treatment of a physical or mental health condition of any individual that proximately causes physical or mental harm
- Counseling any individual to disregard the instruction or counsel of a licensed health care professional or to discontinue any treatment prescribed or recommended by a licensed health care professional
- Counseling any individual to discontinue the use of legend drugs or therapeutic devices prescribed to the individual by a licensed health care professional authorized to prescribe such drugs or devices
- Administering, prescribing, possessing for sale, selling or dispensing any legend drug or medical oxygen
- Indicating in any way that the practitioner is licensed by the State
- Performing or providing enteral or parenteral nutrition
- Promising a cure
- Setting a fracture of a bone
- Delivering a baby
- Providing or performing an abortion
- Inserting intra uterine devices
- Providing complementary or alternative services to either of the following persons without the consent of a parent or legal guardian: a person who is less than 18 years of age or a person that is known to be mentally incompetent

Myths about Exemption Bills

Myth #1 The legalization of all of these professions will create a regulatory nightmare.

Experience shows otherwise. Minnesota passed its law in 2000. There were only 31 investigations during the first four years after the law passed, all for violations everyone would agree warrant investigation – engaging in prohibited activities, sexual misconduct, etc.

When Boards can only investigate practitioners for doing something wrong, they have less, not more, to do.

Myth #2 The availability of alternative care may cause some people to postpone necessary, traditional care.

The term "necessary" is open to interpretation, and actually should be left up to the individual. In fact, research shows that many "necessary" traditional treatments are not very effective, as you have learned in this book. People should have the right to make their own decisions, and to decline traditional treatment if they want to.

Myth #3 In order to protect public health, unlicensed practitioners should be kept out of business.

There is no evidence to support this statement. But, every day people *are* harmed by FDA approved drugs prescribed by licensed professionals. Vioxx is a good example – this was an FDA-approved drug that was dispensed by many licensed medical doctors. The FDA's own representative, Dr. David Graham, estimates that 58,000 people died as a result of taking it. This clearly demonstrates that licensure does not guarantee safety.

In fact, legalizing non-licensed practitioners would *enhance* public safety for the following reasons:

- Practitioners would be able to legally take patient histories before making recommendations about supplements and other natural remedies. This is important since practitioners knowledgeable about herbs and supplements know about drug/nutrient interactions and when certain supplements or foods should be avoided.

- Practitioners could refer clients to medical doctors when appropriate without fear of being reported to a regulatory board.
- Disclosure would be required, so consumers would have some knowledge of the background and training of non-licensed practitioners prior to the delivery of services

Myth #4 Non-licensed practitioners should have their own standards of practice, and their own governing board.

This is unnecessary and impractical. First, there are too many modalities, and the educational pathways are quite diverse. For example, reiki, Rolfing, reflexology, polarity, shiatsu, healing touch, alphabiotics, and cranio-sacral work are all forms of bodywork. But, each type of practitioner is trained in a different way, so there would be no practical way to consolidate non-licensed body workers into a board that would administer an exam, or develop standards of practice for everyone. We'd have to have a separate board for each modality, which would require another government building just to house all the new boards.

The fact remains that there is very little potential for harm from these types of practices. These non-licensed practices are being performed daily throughout the U.S. by hundreds of thousands of people, and being offered to millions of Americans annually. Wouldn't it be better to have everybody operating legally and above ground with some disclosure required? As long as the public wants these services, and is willing to spend billions of dollars per year to access them, providers will continue to offer them. It's time for the legislature to bring the laws in line with the desires and current practices of citizens.

Myth #5 Alternative practices are available through licensed practitioners.

Although more licensed professionals are developing an interest in alternative modalities, most have limited knowledge of them. This is well-documented in the medical literature. In one study, healthcare professionals scored an average of 50% on an exam regarding herbal supplement knowledge.[246] Registered dietitians scored an average of 63% on a similar exam.[247] Research shows that 55% of physicians are not comfortable discussing Complementary and Alternative practices with their patients.[248]

In fact, during one hearing in front of an Ohio House committee, eighteen consumers testified about their own experience with non-licensed practitioners. Their stories collectively represented decades of medical care administered through dozens of health care practitioners. Not one of those practitioners offered the services that ultimately helped these people to get better, and not one of them referred these patients to a practitioner who offered these services either. In fact, the patients testified that in many instances, their doctors threatened them or tried to dissuade them from seeking alternative care, even though they were not getting better with traditional care.

Myth #6 If these practitioners are practicing and people are receiving services now, there is no need to pass a law.
Many practitioners take the risk of being investigated and prosecuted every day that they offer services. Some practitioners can afford to defend themselves, but most cannot. Therefore, they stay underground. This keeps many of them from earning a living at their trade, and makes it difficult for consumers to find them.

The opponents to Health Freedom bills are generally licensure boards and state associations of licensed professionals. They're usually well-funded and well-organized, and intent on protecting their turf. But there is no question that the number of consumers and practitioners who are interested in medical choice is much larger.

Why Licensure Reform is Needed Now

As you have learned in this book, the messages most Americans receive daily about diet, health, and medical treatment are inaccurate. You also have read that there are many groups and companies interested in making sure that these inaccurate messages continue to be widely distributed – billions of dollars are at stake. One of the ways to maintain control of the content of these messages is to control who is allowed to deliver them, and licensure laws are important tools in accomplishing this goal.

While I agree that education and practice standards are important, our current credentialing and licensing system has allowed people with poor training, economic conflicts of interest, and often terrible track records (poor health outcomes for patients) to be the sole providers of health information and health care.

The logical choice when a system is failing is to change it; it is time to allow new practitioners with new ideas to join the discussion and help solve our mounting health care problems.

Other Consumer Choice Issues

There are many other consumer health issues, including mandatory vaccination schedules, school nutrition, matters of public health policy, employee health and wellness, insurance reimbursement, academic freedom, making effective cancer treatments available in the U.S., and more. In fact, there will be a never-ending list of important health care issues to deal with for decades to come.

A strong, well-funded public policy organization capable of working on these issues on an ongoing basis is needed.

The Wellness Forum Public Policy Institute works on legislative and public policy issues in all states and at the federal level. We provide advice on drafting legislation; guidance on opposing legislation that restricts choice; we help to prepare testimony for hearings; provide experts to deliver testimony; and conduct research in order to prepare and present relevant information to government agencies involved in developing and administering nutrition and health policies.

Our organization has had some success, but our future success depends on recruiting more people to get involved, which has proven to be more challenging than I ever imagined. I regularly talk to people who are not registered to vote, they do not know who their elected officials are, they do not belong to an organization that is fighting these battles, and they provide no financial support for these efforts. This has to change. I firmly believe that the largest special interest group in the U.S. is comprised of citizens who want the freedom to choose their own health care practitioners and to choose their method of health care. These same people would also like for local and federal nutrition and health care policies to be based on the best science available. The problem is that unless we unite and make our voices heard, our elected officials and policy-makers will listen to the groups that are screaming the loudest and spending the most money – the traditional medical profession, pharmaceutical companies, agricultural organizations, and others with a vested interest in the status quo.

This is the time to get involved. The level of dissatisfaction with traditional medicine has never been greater. The desire for people to take control of their own destiny has never been stronger. The ability, through the internet and the media, to get our message out and connect with one another has never been better. Let's seize this opportunity to take our rights back as citizens, to make our own choices about health and to control our own destiny. Let's pool our efforts and remind our elected officials that they work for us and they will be fired if they do not vote as we want them to on these issues. Let's make history by forcing the restructuring of our health care system, which is badly broken. Most important, let's demonstrate to ourselves, to our society, to our children, and to the world, that democracy works and actually does represent the will of the people.

For more information, contact:
The Wellness Forum Public Policy Institute
614 841-7700

Employers Can Help to Improve America's Health

Employers have many reasons for becoming catalysts for health care reform. They are currently paying a staggering amount of money to provide health benefits to their employees, and the costs are increasing at an alarming rate.

While companies spend more and more on health insurance, employees get sicker and sicker. This not only increases the cost of benefits, but job performance suffers as well. People don't think well when they don't feel well. They do less when they are tired. Sick people are more prone to accidents, and unhealthy people miss more days of work, which interrupts workflow and decreases productivity. And many unhealthy employees have unhealthy family members, like sick children, who cause their parents to miss work as well.

The current system reinforces the problem. Business owners are still paying most, and some of them all, of the cost of health insurance. Family coverage is offered to employees of almost all large companies. Employees are reimbursed for sick care, but there generally is no reward for maintaining good health (although healthier people *are* rewarded with a longer and better quality of life!).

Employees generally have little financial accountability for the rising costs they are incurring, and the employer usually absorbs the cost of absenteeism and disability due to illness. Inadvertently, we have created a culture in most companies that no one deliberately would have designed. The reward and responsibility structure must change in order for costs to be controlled.

Until recently the main focus for cost-containment has been to reduce benefits, increase the deductible, increase the employee's share of the premiums, and to try to contain the cost of medical services. These approaches are not, however, permanent solutions. There is a limit to how much employees can pay for insurance, and there is a limit to how much benefits can be reduced. Pharmaceutical companies are not going to give away their products, and doctors are working for lower wages than ever before. There will never be enough savings from cost cutting to truly solve the problem.

The best solution, and the one that does permanently solve the problem, is to improve employee health and reduce utilization of medical services.

This approach is different than the "wellness" programs offered by many companies, and sometimes by their insurance providers. While lunchtime workshops, contests, and cooking classes are helpful in raising awareness, they lack accountability and there is little evidence that they actually reduce costs. Programs designed to get people to take their medications on time or check their blood sugar more regularly may be better than nothing, but people stay sick.

Employer health cost reduction programs are designed to reduce costs by using the diet you have learned about in this book to improve employee health. This results in real cost savings.

For example, traditional approaches to treating cardiovascular disease are extremely expensive. The five-year cost of taking care of a patient who has bypass surgery is $100,522.00; for patients undergoing angioplasty it is $81,790.00.[249] Annual costs for statin drugs range from $900 to $1800, not including the cost of physician visits for monitoring and the side effects of the drugs, which are quite common. The cost for Dr. Esselstyn's dietary program which stops the progression of, and sometimes reverses heart disease is only $1500.

The average annual cost for treating a diabetic patient is $11,744.[250] The cost for learning the dietary protocol that reverses most cases of type 2 diabetes taught by The Wellness Forum is less than $500.

According to the Cochrane Collaboration, medications prescribed to treat multiple sclerosis are ineffective and in most cases the side effects and costs outweigh any benefits of taking them. In fact, within 10 years of diagnosis, over 50% of patients are walking with assistance, confined to a wheelchair, or dead, after receiving the best drug treatment medicine has to offer.[251]

Yet the annual cost of these ineffective treatments for patients with MS is approximately $20,000 for drugs and $50,000 for total care.[252] The cost for Dr. McDougall's program, which stops the progression of multiple sclerosis in early-stage patients is a one-time fee of only $4000.

Changing the System

The beginning of change starts with a forward –thinking CEO who decides that not only is it in the best interest of the company and its financial future to change the system, but that it is in the best interest of the employees as well.
The CEO must be willing to tackle the situation in a very comprehensive manner, addressing every way in which the company deals with food, nutrition, and health. This should include paying attention to things like vending machines in the facility, the availability of junk food throughout the day, smoking policies, and food served at company events.

It is important that the company provide tools for helping employees change their health in order to produce results, remembering that if people could do this on their own, they would have done so by now. These tools should include establishing health improvement goals with each employee, educational programming, and rewards and consequences for healthy/unhealthy behaviors. For some companies, an onsite medical doctor and fitness center can be justified. Changes in health care plans to allow for more choice (paying for a physical trainer instead of back surgery, for example) can be valuable in controlling costs. And Health Savings Accounts can make employees much more conscious about the need for and costs of tests and procedures.

The most effective programs involve eventual company-wide participation – in other words, the company pays for the classes and programs, the activities take place on company time, and employees are required to attend.

The goal is to create a culture of health within the company. This takes time. But over time, particularly if everyone is participating, the company's culture can change so that healthy habits are practiced by most, and become the new standard for behavior.

One of the most important keys to success is participation by the company owner and key members of management. I have never seen a health improvement program work when the people in charge didn't participate, and I have personally walked away from potential clients when the CEO and upper management made it clear that they were not on board.

Employer health improvement programs can yield astounding results. Dr. John McDougall conducted a program for Blue Cross/Blue Shield of Minnesota between 1997 and 2001. Three groups of patients were selected based on their high utilization of health care services. These patients participated in an 8-day residential program with one year of follow-up, during which they were taught to consume a plant-based diet similar to the one recommended by The Wellness Forum, and received other forms of lifestyle training.

The results were a *44% annual reduction* in health care costs during a period of time when non-participators experienced a *12% increase* in costs. This translates into a net 56% positive change!

Whole Foods, the largest retailer of organic foods in the world, is now using dietary intervention to address the health issues of its associates and to reduce costs. The company is paying for its associates to attend residential immersion programs at which they learn about the connection between diet and health, and how to adopt a plant-based diet from many of the health care professionals you have read about in this book, including me. The company has committed millions of dollars to this project, and the results, both cost savings and health improvement, are being tracked for publication in medical journals. Visionary Whole Foods co-founder John Mackey is hoping to create a model that other companies will use to improve employee health and reduce costs.

Employers are concerned about the investment required for a health improvement program. The current cost of corporate health plans is extremely high, and rising. Costs will not be reduced without an investment. In fact, the money is going to be spent one way or another – continued increased costs of supporting the current sick care system within the company, or

284

the costs of changing employees' health status so that eventually those costs an be reduced. The obvious, better choice is the latter, and the only way that costs can ultimately be contained.

Corporations are well positioned to educate people about the importance of achieving and maintaining optimal health, as well as the necessity for taking personal responsibility for one's own health status. Not only will companies that participate in this process realize huge savings, they will also have a more productive workforce, less absenteeism, lower turnover, fewer accidents, and a better work environment.

The Wellness Forum offers many comprehensive and effective cost reduction programs for employers. For more information visit www.wellnessforum.com or call 614 841-7700.

Improving School Food and Children's Health

The School Lunch Program:
a Brief History

Congress authorized the school lunch program after World War II to bolster child nutrition, prevent poor childhood health and ***expand the market for surplus foods produced by farmers.*** This dual mission represents a conflict of interest – the best diet for children does not include many of the surplus foods produced by farmers. The program is administered by the USDA, which is already burdened with a conflict of interest in both representing America's farmers and developing dietary guidelines for Americans.

From the beginning, the school lunch program was subsidized by the federal government, but in the early 1980's due to budget constraints, federal subsidies were reduced from 39% of the cost of a meal to 13%. As a result, school lunch prices increased, and more children brought lunch to school. Some schools discontinued their lunch programs and others added a la carte items to increase profitability.

By 1996 only 50% of low-income children and 46% of middle-to upper-income children were buying school lunches. In response, standards were relaxed to allow schools to "entice" kids to purchase lunch at school.

Schools only had to comply with federal dietary guidelines on the federally subsidized portion of lunch, while revenue-generating a la carte items did not have to comply with any standards at all. This opened the door for lots of unhealthy options, junk foods in vending machines, and even fast food outlets in schools.

The guidelines for school lunches have never been ideal. Lunches must contain 1/3 of the daily requirement for protein, Vitamin A, Vitamin C, iron, calcium and calories. The calorie requirement alone is a problem – most kids are eating more than three meals per day, so consuming 1/3 of the total calories for the day at lunchtime contributes to weight gain. Guidelines for fat consumption are quite liberal; the upper limit is 30%, with no more than 10% allowed from saturated fat.

Food service directors are allowed two options for meal planning, the food group standard or nutrient standard. Although this has changed in many schools, most schools still use the food group standard, which requires, among other things, that dairy is served with every meal.

Budgets in school cafeterias are tight. Schools in compliance with these guidelines receive: $ .24 for each meal purchased by a student, $2.17 for reduced price lunches, and $2.57 for fully subsidized government meals provided to children

Food service directors are often blamed for the poor nutritional quality of meals, but many of them are simply responding to economic realities, USDA requirements, and the delivery of unhealthy commodity foods like cheese and meat by the government for use in cafeterias.

But lunches are the not the only way in which kids get access to unhealthy foods at school. In grade school, kids bring cake, ice cream, and other treats for birthday parties. Most schools have vending machines in which soft drinks and junk foods are made available. School stores, athletic events, fundraisers and holiday celebrations are usually opportunities for kids to access high-calorie, sugar- and fat-laden foods.

In fact, according to a 2000 Report from the USDA:
- 77.7% of all middle/senior high schools have vending machines that are accessible by students
- Foods sold as fundraisers compete with school meals in 25.3% of middle schools and 41.6% of high schools
- Milk, fruit juice, ice cream, and cookies are the most common a la carte sellers in elementary schools
- Fruit drinks, pizza, snacks, chips, ice cream, cookies and French Fries are top a la carte sellers in middle/secondary schools

According to a study of students in 13 schools who purchased 10,219 snacks in one week:
- 88.5% of snacks sold in student stores were high in fat
- The average sugar content was 23 grams per snack

290

●Not one fresh fruit or vegetable was sold as a snack in these schools during the week in which data were collected[253]

It's clear that things need to change, but there are many objections to overcome. Some school administrators state that children's nutrition is not their problem. But I contend that it is. Nutrition is taught in school, and food is served in school. When the schools stop including nutrition education in the curriculum and serving meals at school, it will no longer be their problem.

Another argument is that kids are going to eat junk food anyway, so schools should not be burdened with restricting it on campus. But this argument is ridiculous and inconsistent with the approach used to deal with other issues. For example, many kids experiment with alcohol, but I don't know anyone that this is a justification for making it available at school.

Some argue that kids won't eat healthy foods, and that schools cannot afford to lose the revenue from vending machines. But research has shown that kids will choose healthy foods, even when unhealthy choices are available, if they are provided with the right education. And many schools have changed selections in vending machines without negatively affecting revenues.

In fact, often the revenues from vending machines are overestimated and do not take into account revenues lost from other operations. A 2003 Texas Department of Agriculture Survey showed that revenue from vending machines from all 1256 schools was $51 million. But food service departments lost close to $60 million in federal reimbursement for meals which was attributed to sales of competing foods, some of which were purchased in vending machines. The survey concluded that a deficit of $23.7 million resulting from vending operations was being subsidized by the school system.[254]

Administrators at low-performing schools often state that problems other than food are more pressing, while administrators at higher-performing schools tend to think they don't need to pay attention to nutrition because the kids are doing well academically.

Both are wrong. According to the *Student Health Risk, Resilience, and Academic Performance in California Study*, "... health risk and low resilience assets typically have equally detrimental consequences for subsequent test score gains in low- and high-performing schools."

This survey further concluded that "California schools with high percentage of students who routinely engage in some physical activity and healthy eating experience greater subsequent gains in test score than other schools." The report also stated, "Two types of inadequate nutrition – undernourishment and skipping breakfast – have deleterious consequences for subsequent gains in test scores."

All schools are concerned with academic achievement. And studies show that weight and health affect academics. Severely overweight children and adolescents are 4 times more likely than healthy-weight children to report "impaired school functioning."[255]

Overweight children are more likely to have abnormal scores on the Child Behavior Checklist, and are 2 times more likely to be placed in special education and remedial classes than normal weight kids.[256]

This just makes common sense, but poor nutritional status and hunger interfere with cognitive function and lower academic achievement.[257]

Overweight children are more likely to miss school because they are more likely to develop conditions like asthma, type-2 diabetes, depression and anxiety, and sleep apnea.[258]

With your help, we can improve both the quality of food served in our schools and the health of our kids. Anyone can help – parents, teachers, school nurses, school administrators, food service directors and employees, and interested community members.

Start talking to others and build a coalition of people who are interested in working on these issues. If your school has a nutrition or wellness committee, join and offer to help. If your school does not have such a committee, offer to help form one.

Let The Wellness Forum Foundation help you. The foundation is a 501 (c) 3 organization committed to improving children's health throughout the U.S. The foundation provides several services that can help you in your local school or school system, including:

- Free nutrition education for classroom teachers based on Wellness Forum programming
- Free non-industry sponsored classroom materials for teachers who complete our educational program.
- Free assistance in developing sound school nutrition policies
- Free assistance in developing and implementing plans for changing foods served in the cafeteria

Fortunately, there are a growing number of schools who have made significant changes in the nutritional quality of foods served to students. These programs have been proven to work both financially and logistically and provide wonderful models to use in other schools.

For more information about how you can become involved with The Wellness Forum Foundation, visit www.wellnessforumkids.org or call 614 841-7700.

Why Diet-Centered Health Care is Best
For America and the World

> "...While patients are grateful for new drugs and operations,
> what they really want
> is not to be patients at all.
> In this we are failing them."
> David Barker, M.D.

For many decades, the practice of medicine has expanded to include more and more diagnostic tests, more drugs and procedures, and increasingly sophisticated technology, in an attempt to diagnose disease at its earliest stages and improve treatment ourtcomes. The reality is this enormous investment of money and other resources has not paid off.   Early detection has not resulted in a decreased death rate for most degenerative conditions, and most of the drugs and procedures commonly used are ineffective or dangerous.

While the medical system has failed to solve our health problems, Americans have developed some erroneous beliefs about the cause of disease, and the power of the medical system to cure it. Many believe that their health status is outside of their control, and influenced by genes, or even just bad luck. People tend to become concerned with their health when they have been diagnosed with an illness, rather than working to keep themselves healthy. Diagnostic testing often sends the wrong message; people think a clean bill of health gives them permission to continue their less-than-optimal habits.

Once people develop an illness, they generally do not expect to re-gain their health. Most patients don't even ask health care professionals about their track record in stopping the progression of disease or reversing it. If they did most doctors who respond honestly would reply that stopping or reversing disease is not possible. The best that can be expected from drugs and surgery is to slow the progression of disease; unfortunately, standard medical care usually results in patients continuing to get worse and needing more drugs and procedures.

Americans do not tolerate these types of poor results in most other aspects of their lives. For example, think about this concept as it relates to taking care of your car. Imagine taking your car to a garage because the brakes are squeaking and asking the store manager about the store's track record in fixing brakes. What would you do if the store manager replied, "Brakes cannot be fixed. If you bring the car in every few months, we can make sure you don't hit the trees and mailboxes as fast, but we simply cannot fix brakes." You would not leave the car or agree to pay for such work, but Americans settle for similar incompetence every day when they hire most traditional health care practitioners.

The United States is going bankrupt paying for this mostly ineffective care. Discussions about health care usually start with agreement – we are spending too much and we're getting too little; but they quickly degenerate into heated disagreement when the discussion about how to solve these problems begins.

While evidence continues to mount that traditional approaches to health care are not effective, the body of evidence indicating that the right diet can restore health continues to increase.

The science is clear – a well structured plant-based diet can prevent, stop the progression of, and often even reverse the common degenerative conditions that are destroying the health, quality of life, and finances of many Americans. What is most remarkable is that the cost of adopting this diet is so inexpensive that if every American learned about the proper diet through private lessons based on the fees we charge at The Wellness Forum, the cost would be a little over $462 billion dollars, a fraction of what we are spending on health care annually in the U.S. The government and private industry could afford to underwrite the cost of this education for every man, women and child[259] in the country and still spend less money than we are spending on our current system.

Some might think that the idea of solving such huge problems with diet alone is just too good to be true. But it is true. And once this information becomes common knowledge, the world we live in will become a different place. Degenerative disease will be rare. People will enjoy great health and live their lives fully. The cruelty inflicted on animals through factory farming will become a thing of the past, and the destruction of our environment will be greatly reduced. This is the world I want to live in, and the world I want to leave for my children and grandchildren.

What's Next?

> "You must be the change you wish to see in the world."
> Mahatma Gandhi

As Margaret Mead said, "Never doubt that a small, group of thoughtful, committed citizens can change the world. Indeed, it is the only thing that ever has."

According to author Malcolm Gladwell, "The Tipping Point is that magic moment when an idea, trend or social behavior crosses a threshold, tips and spreads like wildfire."

If you are ready to help plant-based nutrition and a new vision for healthcare to "spread like wildfire," the first step is to begin practicing dietary excellence™ yourself. Leading by example is the most powerful way to influence others.

I strongly advise you to join the Wellness Forum, take our Wellness 101 course, and participate in our ongoing programs. Most people need help in making the transition to an optimal diet, and support in maintaining it.

Share this book with family members and friends. Most people find that the best way to convince others is to provide well-documented information, and then to let them decide for themselves how to respond to it.

Tell your health care providers about your new eating plan and let them see the positive changes in your health. Seeing is believing, and there are many great doctors, nurses and dietitians who are interested in learning about protocols that can help patients to experience better outcomes.

Teach the children in your life about healthy eating. The next generation faces even greater health challenges if we do not intervene. Children love to be involved in choosing foods and cooking – make nutrition and food preparation fun. Introduce them to healthy foods at a young age, and they will benefit for the rest of their lives.

Vote with your checkbook. Remember that every time you purchase *anything*, you are supporting *something*. Look at the foods you purchase, the health care decisions you make, and even the donations you make to charities and determine if these are consistent with your belief system about health and nutrition.

Get involved! There are so many things we all can do to help change the system, ranging from teaching cooking classes at your local recreation center to working on improving school food. The Wellness Forum is always looking for people who want to teach our programs to others, to get involved in public policy work and other important activities that can help reform the system.

The "magic moment" referenced by Gladwell is upon us; we live in an era where information about the power of plant-based nutrition can travel fast; and millions of people are looking for better alternatives for their weight and health issues. We have every reason to believe that with your help, the revolution in health that has already begun will continue to gather more momentum every day.

Resources

Dr. Pam Popper's E-Newsletter

It's free and includes articles on health, editorials, answers to questions from readers, and announcements of upcoming events. To receive the newsletter, send an email with your first and last name and email address to pampopper@msn.com.

Wellness Forum Membership

Membership includes:
- Wellness 101 – a ten-hour course during which you will learn basic principles of health and wellness and the skills necessary to practice dietary excellence and optimal habits. Includes a curriculum book, DVD's, and teleconference classes during which the material is reviewed and questions can be answered.
- Workshops and conference calls on a variety of topics ranging from cooking classes to cancer prevention
- Access to a members-only website featuring recipes, a growing library of educational videos, book reviews and other health-related materials
- Ongoing support to help you in filtering and making sense out of the enormous amount of information about health appearing in the media

Employer Health Cost Reduction Programs

The Wellness Forum offers many comprehensive programs that can reduce health insurance costs for your company. All programs are custom-designed, taking into consideration your company's culture and unique circumstances, and have been proven to reduce health care costs.

The Wellness Forum Institute for Health Studies, Inc.

Certified through the Ohio State board of Career Colleges
Registration number 09-09-1908T

The Wellness Forum Institute for Health Studies is the first school in the U.S. that offers a curriculum based on rigorous science and research proving that a plant-based diet is effective for achieving and maintaining optimal health. Programs are offered for health professionals interested in a diet-centered approach to health care; and those who are interested in alternative educational pathways for becoming healthcare professionals.

The Diet and Lifestyle Intervention Course is designed to teach health care professionals how to use diet and lifestyle as a preventive and curative tool. The program is designed to teach doctors and other health and fitness professionals how to use diet and lifestyle as a preventive and curative tool and how to develop a profitable practice around this philosophy. In addition to diet, issues like vaccinations, diagnostic testing, joint and back injuries, and mental health are covered.

The faculty includes Dr. T. Colin Campbell, Dr. Caldwell Esselstyn Jr., Dr. Neal Barnard. Dr. John McDougall, Dr. Ralph Moss, Dr. Pam Popper, Dr. Larry Palevsky, Dr. Mark Scholtz, William Lessler, and Dr. Alan Goldhamer. Specific protocols are taught as part of the course.

The course is taught via virtual classroom, or conference call. Prior to each call, participants are instructed to read the texts and are emailed copies of the instructor's slides. The calls are interactive and the participants can ask questions at any time.

The Nutrition Educator Diploma Program is for individuals who want a career in a nutrition-related field and are seeking an alternative to traditional dietetics. This program requires that students complete basic science courses that are more rigorous than those required for many undergraduate nutrition degrees; includes courses that combine nutritional science with strategies for assisting clients in achieving and maintaining optimal health and effective approaches for common degenerative conditions; includes many classes designed to teach practical skills needed for gainful employment; and concludes with 200 hours of practical experience during which a candidate must demonstrate his/her ability to work effectively in the nutrition education field.

Program Objectives include providing candidates with a rigorous science-based education in nutrition; teaching students how to teach and incorporate dietary interventions for the prevention, treatment or reversal of common diseases; teaching practical skills for making a living in the nutrition field; insuring that students understand public policy issues that affect nutrition and health of the population; and insuring that students understand how to work within their scope of practice, based on their state of residence

Careers With The Wellness Forum

The Wellness Forum offers training and licensure programs that allows individuals to offer our workshops and courses. These opportunities are designed for people who good communicators, are looking for a part-time or full-time career in a health-related field and are passionate about helping others to achieve optimal health.

The Wellness Forum Foundation

The Wellness Forum Foundation offers programming about proper diet and lifestyle choices to teachers, administrators, food service personnel and others involved in educating our children. The Foundation also makes available age-appropriate curriculum materials, foods samples and other materials for classroom use, free assistance in developing sound school nutrition policies, and free assistance in developing and implementing plans for changing foods served in the cafeteria.
Volunteers are needed! Let us know if you are interested in helping with this very important project!

Wellness Forum Foods

Plant-based chefs are no longer a novelty – there are lots of people who have learned to make fabulous vegan dishes – and many are so good that most people don't notice that the food does not contain animal foods. The problem is that many of the dishes produced by these chefs, while made with plant foods, are unhealthy because of the fat content.

Del Sroufe is the best chef in the U.S. at creating dishes that are not only plant-based, but low-fat and oil-free; almost all meals are compliant with programs like the McDougall Program, Dr. Esselstyn's program and many of the other plant-based gurus who are achieving incredible results with their patients.

Del has mastered the art of captivating the new convert to a plant-based diet with mouth-watering dishes that seem like they are just too good to be healthy. *But they are!* Additionally, he has developed a diverse repertoire of hundreds of recipes that guarantee that no one will ever get bored with or tired of the food.

Chef Del has created an extensive menu that appeals to a wide variety of tastes, ranging from comfort foods to unusual ethnic dishes, all of which feature the freshest, organic ingredients. Any menu item can be custom-prepared in consideration of dietary preferences, allergies, and other restrictions. In addition to delivering food to homes and offices daily throughout Central Ohio, most of the menu can be shipped via overnight service throughout the Continental U.S.

To consult with one of our staff or to place an order, please call 614 888-FOOD (3663). You can view the menu online at www.wellnessforumfoods.com.

The Wellness Forum Public Policy Institute

This subsidiary works on legislative and public policy issues in all states and at the federal level. In order to make faster and more sweeping changes in the system, more voters need to get involved. Membership is free; for more information send an email to pampopper@msn.com.

Health Briefs Online

4000+ pages of articles, most with references, on a wide variety of topics, including soy, supplementation, diagnostic testing, drugs, surgeries, treatment protocols, book reviews and more. This body of material represents close to 10 years of the best information from medical journals and other scientific publications. There is a search engine to help you find the topics you are looking for, and the system allows you to either print out the articles or email articles to people.

The Library is designed to be a resource for both consumers to further their own knowledge and for health care professionals to provide information easily to patients in response to questions and concerns.

Additional Educational Materials and Products

Please visit our website at www.wellnessforum.com or call our office at 614 841-7700 to talk to our staff.

EndNotes

1 www.whitehouse.gov

2 http://www.diabetes.org/diabetes-statistics.jsp

3 http://www.cdc.gov/nccdphp/publications/AAG/dhdsp.htm

4 http://www.cdc.gov/media/pressrel/2009/r090727.htm

5 American Cancer Society *Cancer Facts and Figures 2009* Atlanta Georgia 2009

6 http://www.cdc.gov/diabetes/pubs/pdf/ndfs_2007.pdf

7 http://www.cdc.gov/diabetes/pubs/pdf/ndfs_2007.pdf

8 http://www.cdc.gov/nccdphp/publications/AAG/dhdsp.htm

9 American Cancer Society *Cancer Facts and Figures 2009* Atlanta Georgia 2009

10 "New AAP Policy on Lipid Screening and Heart Health in Children." July 7 2008 accessed online May 17 2010 at http://www.aap.org/advocacy/releases/july08lipidscreening.htm

11 Campbell TCC *The China Study* p 106 Ben Bella Books 2004

12 Castelli W, Doyle J, Gordon T, et al. "HDL cholesterol and other lipids in coronary heart disease." *Circulation* May 1977

13 http://www.usda.gov/wps/portal/!ut/p/_s.7_0_A/7_0_1OB?parentna v=ABOUT_USDA&navid=MISSION_STATEMENT&navtype=RT

14 Mudry, Jessica *The Early History of American Nutrition Research"* accessed online at www.sunypress.edu

15 http://www.ers.usda.gov/publications/arb750/arb750b.pdf
16 http://www.ers.usda.gov/publications/arb750/arb750b.pdf

17 http://www.ers.usda.gov/publications/arb750/arb750b.pdf

18 http://www.ers.usda.gov/publications/arb750/arb750b.pdf

19 http://www.pcrm.org/news/health001206.html

[20] Agribusiness PAC Contributions to Federal Candidates 2008 election cycle accessed online at http://www.opensecrets.org/pacs/sector.php?cycle=2008&txt=A01

[21] USDA, milkfat basis

[22] http://www.dairycheckoff.com/DairyCheckoff/AboutUs/HowTheDairy CheckoffWorks/How-The-Dairy-Checkoff-Works

[23] Report to Congress on the National Dairy Promotion and Research Program and the National Fluid Milk Processor Promotion Program July 1, 2003

[24] American Dietetic Association/ADA Foundation 2008 Annual Report accessed online at http://www.eatright.org/uploadFiles/Media/2008_ADA_Annual_Rep ort_FINAL(4).pdf

[25] Accessed online Feb 25, 2009 www.americanheart.org

[26] http://checkmark.heart.org/ProductsByManufacturer

[27] http://www.americanheart.org/presenter.jhtml?q=caldwell+esselstyn &identifier=10000015&submit.x=32&submit.y=5

[28] Doll, R and Peto, R "The Causes of cancer: Quantitative estimates of avoidable risks of cancer in the United States today." *J Natl Cancer Inst* 66 (1981): 1192-1265

[29] Castelli W, Doyle J, Gordon T, et al. "HDL cholesterol and other lipids in coronary heart disease." *Circulation* May 1977

[30] Karjalainen J, Martin JM, Knip M et al, "A bovine albumin peptide as a possible trigger of insulin-dependent Diabetes Mellitus," *New Engl Journ Med.* 327 (1992):302-307

[31] Akerblom HK, Knip M. "Putative environmental factors and Type 1 diabetes." *Diabetes/Metabolism Revs* 14 (1998):31-67

[32] Naik RG and Palmer JP. "Preservation of beta-cell function in Type-1 Diabetes." *Diabetes Rev.* 7 (1999):154-182

33 Malosse D, Perron H, Sasco A, et al. "Correlation Analysis between Bovine Populations, Other Farm Animals, House Pets, and Multiple Sclerosis Prevalence." *Neuroepidemiology* 12 (1993):15-27

34 Bernstein JM. "The role of IgE-mediated hypersensitivity in the development of otitis media with effusion." *Otolaryngol Clin North Am.* 1992 Feb;25(1):197-211.

35 Juntti H, Tikkanen S, Kokkonen J, Alho OP, Niinimaki A. "Cow's milk allergy is associated with recurrent otitis media during childhood." *Acta Otolaryngol.* 1999;119(8):867-73.

36 Chan JM and Giovannucci EL. "Dairy products, calcium and vitamin D and risk of prostate cancer." *Epidemiol. Revs.* 23 (2001):87-92

37 Facts About Obesity in the United States. Centers for Disease Control and Prevention. National Center for Health Marketing. http://www.cdc.gov/PDF/Facts_About_Obesity_in_the_United_State s.pdf. Nov 2009

38 CDC Weekly Morbidity and Mortality Report October 31, 2008 Karen Kirtland

39 Gottlieb, Scott. "Updates for US Heart Disease Death Rates." *BMJ* 1999 Jan 9; 318(7176):79

40 The ERS Food Consumption (Per Capita)Data System, available at: www.ers.usda.gov/data/foodconsumption/

41 Schulz L, Bennett MB, Ravussin E, Kidd, J, Kidd K, Esparza J, Valencia, M. "Effects of Traditional and Western Environments on Prevalence of Type 2 Diabetes in Pima Indians in Mexico and the U.S." doi: 10.2337/dc06-0138 *Diabetes Care* August 2006 vol. 29 no. 8 1866-1871

42 Schulz L, Bennett MB, Ravussin E, Kidd, J, Kidd K, Esparza J, Valencia, M. "Effects of Traditional and Western Environments on Prevalence of Type 2 Diabetes in Pima Indians in Mexico and the U.S." doi: 10.2337/dc06-0138 *Diabetes Care* August 2006 vol. 29 no. 8 1866-1871

[43] Newman, B, Mu H, Butler LM et al, "Frequency of breast cancer attributable to BRCA1 in a population-based series of American women." *JAMA* 279 (1998):915-921

[44] Cancer Statistics 2009: A Presentation from the American Cancer Society, accessed online at www.cancer.org

[45] Wu, A.H., Pike M.C. and Stram D.O. "Meta analysis: dietary fat intake, serum estrogen levels and the risk of breast cancer." *J. Natl. Cancer Inst.* 91 (1999):529-534

[46] Haenszel W and Kurihara M. "Studies of Japanese migrants: mortality from cancer and other disease among Japanese and the United States." *J. Natl. Cancer Inst.* 40 (1968):43-68

[47] Armstrong B, Doll R. Environmental factors and cancer incidence and mortality in different countries, with special reference to dietary practices. *Int J Cancer* 1975;15:617-31
.

[48] Lands WEM, Hamazaki T, Yamazaki K, et al. Changing dietary patterns. *Am J Clin Nutr* 1990;51:991-3.

[49] M Knip et al, "Environmental Triggers and Determinants of Type 1 Diabetes." *Diabetes* 54, suppl 2 (December 2005):S125-36

[50] Haas, C, Creighton, C, Pi, X, et al. "Identification of genes modulated in rheumatoid arthritis using complementary DNA microarray analysis of lymphoblastoid B cell lines from disease-discordant monozygotic twins"*Arthritis and Rheumatism*, Vol. 54, No. 7, July 2006, pp 2047-2060.

[51] Keys A, Menotti A, Karvonen M, et al. The diet and 15-year death rate in the Seven Countries Study. *Am J Epidemiol.* 1986;124:903–915

[52] Garcia-Closas R, Berenguer A, González CA."Changes in food supply in Mediterranean countries from 1961 to 2001." Public Health Nutr. 2006 Feb;9(1):53-60

[53] World Health Organization Global Obesity Report

[54] Vrentos, G, Papadakis J, Malliaraki N, et al. "Diet serum homocysteine levels and ischaemic heart disease in a Mediterranean population" British Journal of Nutrition, Volume 91, Issue 06, Jun

2004, pp 1013-1019 doi: 10.1079/BJN20041145 (About doi), Published online by Cambridge University Press 09 Mar 2007

55 Lorgeril, et al, "Mediterranean Diet, Traditional Risk Factors, and the Rate of Cardiovascular Complications After Myocardial Infarction: Final Report of the Lyon Diet Heart Health Study," *Circulation* Feb 16, 1999

56 Allen, et al, "A prospective study of diet and prostate cancer in Japanese men," *Cancer Causes Control* 2004;15:911-20

57 Virtanen, et al, "Mercury, fish oils and risk of acute coronary events and cardiovascular disease, coronary heart disease and all-cause mortality in men in eastern Finland," *Arterioscler Thromb Vasc Biol* 2005;25:228-33

58 Lee Hooper, et al Risks and benefits of omega 3 fats for mortality, cardiovascular disease, and cancer: systematic review *BMJ.* 2006 April 1; 332(7544): 752–760. doi: 10.1136/bmj.38755.366331.2F.

59 Blankenhorn, D.H. et al, "The Influence of Diet on the Appearance of New Lesions in Human Coronary Arteries." *JAMA* March 23, 1990. 263(12):1646-1652.

60 Rudel, Lawrence L, et al "Compared with Dietary Monounsaturated and Saturated Fat, Polyunsaturated Fat Protects African Green Monkeys from Coronary Artery Arteriosclerosis." *Arteriosclerosis, Thrombosis, and Vascular Biology* December 1995

61 Vogel, R. et al, "The Postprandial Effect of Components of the Mediterranean Diet on Endothelial Function." *J Am Coll Card* 2000

62 Felton C. et al. "Dietary polyunsaturated fatty acids and composition of human aortic plaques" *Lancet*, 1994, 344:1195

63 B Hennig and BA Watkins "Linoleic acid and linolenic acid: effect on permeability properties of cultured endothelial cell monolayers." *Am J Clin Nutr* 1989 49: 301-305

64 Lone Frost Larsen; Else-Marie Bladbjerg; Jørgen Jespersen; ; Peter Marckmann "Effects of Dietary Fat Quality and Quantity on Postprandial Activation of Blood Coagulation Factor VII." *Arteriosclerosis, Thrombosis, and Vascular Biology.* 1997;17:2904-2909.

309

[65] USDA "What's in the Foods You Eat" Search Tool 11/9/2009

[66] Hegsted DM.. " Minimum protein requirements of adults." *Am J Clin Nutr.* 1968 May; 21(5): 352-7.

[67] Prentice A "Constituents of Human Milk" United Nations University Centre

[68] Chittenden, R. H. (1904). Physiological economy in nutrition, with special reference to the minimal protein requirement of the healthy man. An experimental study. New York: Frederick A. Stokes Company.

[69] source nutritiondata.com accessed 11/26/2009

[70] Campbell, C *The China Study* BenBella Books 2005 p 78

[71] Report delivered by Dr. David Graham to a Senate Finance Committee chaired by Senator Grassley November 18, 2004

[72] Neal D. Barnard, M.D. et al "A Low-Fat Vegan Diet Elicits Greater Macronutrient Changes But is Comparable in Adherence and Acceptability Compared with a More Conventional Diabetes Diet Among Individuals With Type 2 Diabetes." *J Am Dietetic Assoc* Feb 2009; vol 109 no 2:263-272

[73] Barnard, Neal, et al, "Adherence and Acceptability of a Low-Fat Vegetarian Diet Among Patients With Cardiac Disease," *Jrnl of Cardiopulmonary Rehab.* Vol 12, no 6; Nov-Dec 1992

[74] Bjelakovic G, Nikolova D, Gluud LL, Simonetti RG, Gluud C. Antioxidant supplements for prevention of mortality in healthy participants and patients with various diseases. Cochrane Database of Systematic Reviews 2008, Issue 2. Art. No.: CD007176. DOI: 10.1002/14651858.CD007176.

[75] Greenberg, ER, Joan A. Baron, JA, Tostenson, TD et al, "A Clinical Trial of Antioxidant Vitamins to Prevent Colorectal Adenoma." *New Engl J Med* vol. 331, no. 3 July 21 1994: 141-147

[76] Sesso, Howard, D. et al, "Vitamins C and E in the Prevention of Cardiovascular Disease in Men: The Physicians' Health Study II Randomized Controlled Trial," *JAMA* 2008;300(18):2123-2133

77 Lange H, Suryapranata H, De Luca G, et al. "Folate Therapy and In-Stent Restenosis after Coronary Stenting" *New Eng J Med* June 24, 2004 no 26: vol. 350:2673-2681

78 Albert, CM, et al, "Effects of Folic Acid and B vitamins on Risk of Cardiovascular Events and Total Mortality Among Women at High Risk for Cardiovascular Disease: A Randomized Trial," *JAMA* vol 299, issue 17, pages 2027-203

79 Lippman SM, Klein EA, Goodman PJ, Lucia MS, et al. "Effect of selenium and vitamin E on risk of prostate cancer and other cancers: the Selenium and Vitamin E Cancer Prevention Trial (SELECT)." *JAMA*. 2009 Jan 7;301(1):39-51. Epub 2008 Dec 9.

80 http://www.iom.edu/Reports/2010/Dietary-Reference-Intakes-for-Calcium-and-Vitamin-D/Report-Brief.aspx

81 Freedman, D.Michal, et al, "Prospective Study of Serum Vitamin D and Cancer Mortality in the U.S.," *J Natl Canc Inst* Oct 30 2007; 99(21):1594-1602; doi 10:1093

82 Avenell, A, Cook J, MacLennan G, McPherson G. "Vitamin D Supplementation and Type 2 Diabetes: A Substudy of a Randomised Placebo-controlled Trial in Older People." *Ageing*. 2009;38(5):606-609.

83 *Alternative Therapies* May/June 2008 vol 14 no 3

84 Tuohimaa P, Tenkanen L, Ahonen M, Lumme S, et al. "Both high and low levels of blood vitamin D are associated with a higher prostate cancer risk: a longitudinal, nested case-control study in the Nordic countries." *Int J Cancer*. 2004 Jan 1;108(1):104-8.

85 Heikkinen AM, Tuppurainen MT, Komulainen M, et al. "Long-term vitamin D3 supplementation may have adverse effects on serum lipids during postmenopausal hormone replacement therapy." *Eur J Endocrinol* 1997;137:495-502.

86 Jacobus CH, Holick MF, Shao Q, Chen TC, Holm IA, Kolodny JM, Fuleihan GE, Seely EW. "Hypervitaminosis D associated with drinking milk." *N Engl J Med*. 1992 Apr 30;326(18):1173-7

87 Lee RD, Nieman DC. Nutrition Assessment, 2nd edition. St. Louis, MO Mosby 1996

[88] Key T, Appleby P, Spencer E, Travis, R, Roddam A, Allen N. "Mortality in British vegetarians: results from the European Prospective Investigation into Cancer and Nutrition." *Am J Clin Nutr* (March 18, 2009). doi:10.3945/ajcn.2009.26736L

[89] Lan T Ho-Pham, Nguyen D Nguyen, and Tuan V Nguyen "Effect of vegetarian diets on bone mineral density: a Bayesian meta-analysis."*Am. J. Clinical Nutrition*, Oct 2009; 90: 943 – 950

[90] Hiller T, Stone, K, Bauer D, et al. "Evaluating the Value of Repeat Bone Mineral Density Measurement and Prediction of Fractures in Older Women." *Arch Intern Med.* 2007;167(2):155-160.

[91] Boffeta, P, Couto, E, Wichman J, et al. "Fruit and Vegetables Intake and Overall Cancer Risk in the European Prospective Investigation into Cancer and Nutrition." *JNCI* published online April 6 2010; doi:10.1093/jnci/djq072

[92] Esselstyn, CB. Ellis SG, Mendendorp SV et al. "A strategy to arrest and reverse coronary artery disease: a 5-year longitudinal study of a single physician's practice." *J Family Practice* 41 (1995):560-568
[93] Esselstyn CJ. "Introduction: more than coronary artery disease." *Am J Cardiol.* 83 (1998):5T-9T

[94] Swank RL. "Effect of low saturated fat diet in early and late cases of multiple sclerosis." *Mancer* 336 (1990):91-103

[95] Campbell, TCC, *The China Study* Ben Bella Books 2004 pp 51-67

[96] Kenneth K Carroll "Dietary Fats and Cancer." *Am J Clin Nutr* 1991;53:1064S-7S

[97] Chan JM and Giovannucci EL. "Dairy products, calcium and vitamin D and risk of prostate cancer." *Epidemiol. Revs.* 23 (2001):87-92

[98] Lee RD, Nieman DC. Nutrition Assessment, 2nd edition. St. Louis, MO Mosby 1996

[99] Zemel MB, Thompson W, Milstead A, Morris K, Campbell P. "Calcium and dairy acceleration of weight and fat loss during energy restriction in obese adults." *Obes Res.* 2004;12: 582–90.

[100] Zemel MB, Shi H, Greer B, DiRienzo D, Zemel PC. "Regulation of adiposity by dietary calcium." *FASEB J.* 2000;14: 1132–8.

[101] Lanou, Amy Joy; Barnard, Neal D "Dairy and weight loss hypothesis: an evaluation of the clinical trials." *Nutrition Reviews*, Volume 66, Number 5, May 2008 , pp. 272-279(8)

[102] Berkey C, Rockett HRH, Willett W, Colditz G. "Milk, Dairy Fat, Dietary Calcium, and Weight Gain A Longitudinal Study of Adolescents." *Arch Pediatr Adolesc Med.* 2005;159:543-550.

[103] http://www.acsh.org/healthissues/newsID.1140/healthissue_detail.asp

[104] http://www.acsh.org/healthissues/newsID.1140/healthissue_detail.asp

[105] http://www.acsh.org/healthissues/newsID.1140/healthissue_detail.asp

[106] Mindfully.org. 01/08/2004 Accessed at http://www.mindfully.org/Pesticide/ACSH-koop.htm

[107] http://www.medicalnewstoday.com/articles/29838.php

[108] Breven, et al, "Physician disclosure of healthy personal behaviors improves credibility and ability to motivate" *Archives of Family Medicine* 2000 Mar:9(3):287-90)

[109] Strom A, Jensen R. Mortality from circulatory disease in Norway 1940." *Lancet* 1951 Jan 20; 1(6647):126-9

[110] Prochazka, A, Lundahl, K, Pearson, W et al. "Support of Evidence-Based Guidelines for the Annual Physical Examination: a Survey of Primary Care Providers." *Arch Intern Med.* 2005;165:1347-1352

[111] Olsen O; Gotzsche PC "Cochrane review on screening for breast cancer with mammography." *Lancet* 2001 Oct 20;358(9290):1340-2

[112] Thomas H. Lee, M.D> et al, "Screening For Prostate Cancer." *N Engl J Med* March 26,2009; no 13 vol 360:e18

[113] Fritz H. Schroder, M.D> et al "Screening and Prostate-Cancer Mortality in a Randomized European Study." *N Engl J Med* March 26, 2009; no 13 vol 360:1320-1328

[114] Eleven-year survival in the Veterans Administration randomized trial of coronary bypass surgery for stable angina. The Veterans Administration Coronary Artery Bypass Surgery Cooperative Study Group. *New Engl J Med* 1984 Nov 22;311(2):1333-1339

[115] Varnauskas A "Twelve year follow-up of survival in the randomized European Coronary Surgery Study." *New Engl J Med* Aug 11 1988 vol 319:332-337

[116] Fisher B, Costantino JP, Wickerham DL, et al. Tamoxifen for prevention of breast cancer: Report of the National Surgical Adjuvant Breast and Bowel Project P–1 study. *Journal of the National Cancer Institute* 1998; 90(18):1371–1388.

[117]
http://www.gerber.com/AllStages/About/Press_Room_Detail.aspx?PressId=cc6a607b-efdd-4e93-8b0d-c65e8d94a414

[118] Skinner A, Steiner M, Henderson F, Perrin E. "Multiple Markers of Inflammation and Weight Status: Cross Sectional Analyses Through Childhood." *Pediatrics* published online March 1, 2010 doi10.1542/peds 2009-2182

[119] Belluck, Pam, "Child Obesity Seen as Warning of Heart Disease" *New York Times*, November 12 2009

[120] Ogden C, Carroll, M, Curtin L et al. "Prevalence of Overweight and Obesity in the U.S. 1999-2004." *JAMA* 2006 295:1549-1555

[121]
(http://www.cdc.gov/nchs/products/pubs/pubd/hestats/overweight/overwght_child_under02.htm, NHANES, NCHS).

[122] Luma G, Spiotta R. "Hypertension and Children and Adolescents." *Am Fam Physicians* 2006 May 1; 73 (9):1558-1568

[123] Karjalainen J, Martin JM, Knip M et al, "A bovine albumin peptide as a possible trigger of insulin-dependent Diabetes Mellitus," *New Engl Journ Med.* 327 (1992):302-307

[124] Akerblom HK, Knip M. "Putative environmental factors and Type 1 diabetes." *Diabetes/Metabolism Revs* 14 (1998):31-67

[125] Naik RG and Palmer JP. "Preservation of beta-cell function in Type-1 Diabetes." *Diabetes Rev.* 7 (1999):154-182

[126] http://www.cspinet.org/new/pdf/food_marketing_to_children.pdf

[127] Cogliano V et al. Carcinogenicity of combined oestrogen progestagen contraceptives and menopausal treatment. Lancet Onc. 2005; 6:552-3.

[128] Yager JD et al. Estrogen Carcinogenesis in Breast Cancer. *NEJM* 2006;354: 270-82.

[129] Smith J, Green J, Berrington de Gonzalez A ET AL. "Cervical cancer and the use of hormonal contraceptives: a systemic review." *The Lancet* April 5 2003; vol 361 (9364):1159-1167

[130] http://www.webmd.com/sex/birth-control/news/20071106/artery-plaque-risk-from-the-pill

[131] http://www.creightonmodel.com/

[132] http://www.billings-centre.ab.ca/

[133] Olsen O; Gotzsche PC "Cochrane review on screening for breast cancer with mammography." *Lancet* 2001 Oct 20;358(9290):1340-2

[134] Jorgensen, K, Zahl, P, Gotzsche P. "Breast cancer mortality in organised mammography screening in Denmark: comparative study." *BMJ* 2010;340:c1241
Published 23 March 2010, doi:10.1136/bmj.c1241

[135] A Berrington de Gonzalez et al, "Estimated Risk of Radiation-Induced Breast Cancer From Mammographic Screening for Young BRCA Mutation Carriers."
J. Natl. Cancer Inst. 2009 101: 205-209; doi:10.1093/jnci/djn440

[136] Fletcher and Elmore, "Mammographic screening for breast cancer," *New Engl J Med April 24 2003;* vol. 348, (17): 1672-80

[137] Ostbye, T, "Elderly women overly screened for cancers with little measurable benefit," *Annals of Family Practice,* Nov 2003

315

[138] U.S. Preventive Services Task Force "Screening For Breast Cancer: U.S. Preventive Services Task Force Recommendation." *Ann Intern Med* November 17, 2009 151:1716-1726

[139] Barnard, et al, "Diet and Sex Hormone Binding Globulin, Dysmenorrhea, and Premenstrual Symptoms," *Obstet Gynecol* 2000;95:245-50

[140] Mennella, JA, "Prenatal and postnatal flavor learning by human infants", *Pediatrics*, 2001 June;107(6):E88

[141] Ebbing, M, Bonaa K, Nygard, O et al. "Cancer Incidence and Mortality After Treatment With Folic Acid and Vitamin B12." *JAMA*. 2009;302(19):2119-2126.

[142] Poston L "The Vitamins in Pre-eclampsia Trial." *The Lancet* (DOI:10.1016/S0140-6736(06)68434-1)

[143] Hartmann, K, Viswananthan M, Palmieri R. "Outcomes of Routine Episiotomy: a systematic review." *JAMA*. 2005;293:2141-2148.

[144] Barnard ND, Scialli AR, Turner-McGrievy G, Lanou AJ, Glass J. The effects of a low-fat, plant-based dietary intervention on body weight, metabolism, and insulin sensitivity. *Am J Med*. 2005;118:991-997.

[145] Moynihan R, Heath I, Henry D. Selling sickness: the pharmaceutical industry and disease mongering. *BMJ* 2002; 324: 886-891

[146] Alix Speigel "How A Bone Disease Grew To Fit The Diagnosis." National Public Radio December 2009

[147] Marshall D, Johnell O, Wedel H. Meta-analysis of how well measures of bone mineral density predict occurrence of osteoporotic fractures. *BMJ* 1996;312:1254-1259.

[148] Cummings, S, Black, D, Thomson D, et al. "Effect of Alendronate on Risk of Fractures in Women with Low Bone Density but Without Vertebral Fractures." *JAMA* 1998;280:2077-2082

[149] Mashiba, Tasuku, et al, "Suppressed Bone Turnover by Bisphospanates Increases Microdamage Accumulation and Reduces Some Biomechanical Properties in Dog Rib," *J Bone Min Res* PRIL 2000:15:613-620 (DOI: 10.1359/BMR.2000.15.4.613)

150 Neviaser, Andrew, et al, "Low Energy Femoral Shaft Fractures Associated with Alendronate Use," *J Orth Trauma* May/June 2008 vol 22 #5

151 Peter Sedghizadeh at al, "Oral bisphosphonate use and the prevalence of osteonecrosis of the jaw: an institutional inquiry." *J Am Dent Assoc* 2009;140:61-66

152 Berkow, Susan et al, "Diet and survival after prostate cancer diagnosis" *Nutrition Reviews* vol 65 #9

153 A. Lophatananon, J. Archer, D. Easton, R. Pocock, D. Dearnaley, et al. "Dietary fat and early-onset prostate cancer risk" British Journal of Nutrition   Published online ahead of print, First View Articles, doi: 10.1017/S0007114509993291

154 Giovannucci, E, et al, "Calcium and fructose intake in relation to risk of prostate cancer," *Cancer Res* 1998:58:442-447

155 Giovannucci, E et al, "A prospective study of calcium intake and fatal prostate cancer," *Cancer Epidemiol Biomarkers Prev* 2006 15(2):203-210

156 Chan, JM "Dairy products, calcium, and prostate cancer risk in the Physicians' Health Study," *Am J Clin Nutr* 2001;74:549-554

157 Lippman, S. Klein E, Goodman PJ et al. "Effect of selenium and vitamin E on risk of prostate cancer and other cancers: the Selenium and Vitamin E Cancer Prevention Trial (SELECT)." *JAMA.* 2009 Jan 7;301(1):39-51. Epub 2008 Dec 9.

158 Sesso, Howard, D. et al, "Vitamins C and E in the Prevention of Cardiovascular Disease in Men: the Physicians' Health Study II Randomized Controlled Trial," *JAMA* 2008;300(18):2123-2133

159 Weinstein, SJ et al, "Serum and dietary vitamin in relation to prostate cancer risk," Cancer Epidermiol Biomarkers Prev; 2007 June 16(6): 1253-9

160 Kobayashi, et al, "Detection of prostate cancer in men with prostate-specific antigen levels of 2.0 to 4.0 ng/ml equivalent to that in men with 4.1 to10.0 mg/ml in a Japanese population," 2004 Apr;63(4):727-731

[161] Coldman, et al, "Trends in prostate cancer incidence and mortality; an analysis of mortality change by screening intensity, " *CMAJ* 2003 Jan 7;168(1):31-35

[162] Eastham, J, Riedel E, Scardino P. et al. "Variation of Serum Prostate-Specific Antigen Levels: An Evaluation of Year-to-Year Fluctuations." *JAMA.* 2003;289:2695-2700.

[163] Lu-Yao G, Albertson P, Moore D. "Outcomes of Localized Prostate Cancer Following Conservative Management." *JAMA.* 2009;302(11):1202-1209.

[164] Ornish, Dean et al: Intensive lifestyle changes may affect the progression of prostate cancer. *The Journal of Urology* Vol. 174:1065, 2005.

[165] Lu-Gao GL, et al, "Survival following primary androgen-based deprivation therapy among men with localized prostate cancer," *JAMA* 2008;300:173-181

[166] Bill-Axelson et al, "Radical Prostatectomy versus watchful waiting in early prostate cancer," N Engl J Med. 2005 May 12;352(19):1977-84

[167] Sanda M, Dunn R, Michalsky J et al. "Quality of Life and Satisfaction with Outcome among Prostate-Cancer Survivors." *NEJM* March 20 2008 (358):1250-1261

[168] Alcaraz, A, Arango, O. "Cancer and Other Risks of Vasectomy." *European Journal of Contraception and Reproductive Health Care* December 1996 vol 1 no 4:311-318

[169] Campbell M, Retik A et al *Campbell's Urology* 1997 Elsevier Health Science

[170] Flegal KM, Carroll MD, Ogden CL, et al. "Prevalence and trends in obesity among U.S. adults, 1999-2000." *JAMA* 288 (2002):1723-1727

[171] National Center for Health Statistics. "Obesity still on the rise, new data show. The U.S. Department of Health and Human Services News Release." October 10 2009. Washington D.C.: 2002. Accessed at www://www.cdc.gov/nchs/releases/02news/obesityonrise/htm

[172] Schwimmer, J, Burwinkle T, Varni J "Health-Related Quality of Life of Severely Obese Children and Adolescents" *JAMA*. 2003;289:1813-1819.

[173] Duncan K. "The effects of high- and low- density diets of satiety, energy intake, and eating time of obese and non-obese subjects." *Am J Clin Nutr* 37:76

[174] The ACCORD Study Group. "Effects f combination lipid therapy in type 2 diabetes mellitus." *NEJM*. Mar 18 2010

[175] Mora S, Ridker PM. "Justification for the Use of Statins in Primary Prevention: an Intervention Trial Evaluating Rosuvastatin (JUPITER)." *Am J Cardiol*. 2006;97(2A):33A-41A

[176] Brown BG, Taylor AJ. "Does ENHANCE diminish confidence in lowering LDL or in ezetimibe?" *NEJM* 2008;358(14):1504-1507

[177] Waters, D. "Aggressive lipid-lowering therapy compared with angioplasty on stable coronary artery disease." *NEJM* December 9, 1999 vol 341:1853-1855 no 24

[178] www.enotalone.com

[179] Braunwald, E. "Shattuck lecture –cardiovascular medicine at the turn of the millennium: triumphs, concerns and opportunities." *New Engl. J. Med*. 337 (1997):1360-1369

[180] American Heart Association. "Heart Disease and Stroke Statistics – 2003 Update." Dallas, TX: American Heart Association 2002

[181] http://www.cdc.gov/nccdphp/publications/AAG/dhdsp.htm

[182] Thompson I, Taqngen C et al. "Erectile dysfunction and subsequent cardiovascular disease." *JAMA* December 21 2005; 294:2996-3002.

[183] Esposito K, Ciotola M, Giugliano F, Maiorino MI, Autorino R, De Sio M, Giugliano G, Nicoletti G, D'Andrea F, and Giugliano D. "Effects of intensive lifestyle changes on erectile dysfunction in men." *J Sex Med* 2009;6:243–250.

[184] American Cancer Society "Cancer Facts and Figures – 1998." Atlanta, GA American Cancer Society, 1998

[185] American Cancer Society *Cancer Facts and Figures 2009* Atlanta Georgia 2009

[186] Kobayashi, et al, "Detection of prostate cancer in men with prostate-specific antigen levels of 2.0 to 4.0 ng/ml equivalent to that in men with 4.1 to10.0 mg/ml in a Japanese population," 2004 Apr;63(4):727-731).

[187] Coldman, et al, "Trends in prostate cancer incidence and mortality; an analysis of mortality change by screening intensity." *CMAJ* 2003 Jan 7;168(1):31-35.

[188] U.S. Preventive Services Task Force "Screening For Breast Cancer: U.S. Preventive Services Task Force Recommendation." *Ann Intern Med* November 17, 2009 151:1716-1726

[189] Laura Esserman, MD, MBA; Yiwey Shieh, AB; Ian Thompson, MD "Rethinking Screening for Breast Cancer and Prostate Cancer" *JAMA*. 2009;302(15):1685-1692.

[190] A Berrington de Gonzalez et al, "Estimated Risk of Radiation-Induced Breast Cancer From Mammographic Screening for Young BRCA Mutation Carriers." *J. Natl. Cancer Inst.* 2009 101: 205-209; doi:10.1093/jnci/djn440

[191] American Cancer Society *Cancer Facts and Figures 2009,* Atlanta Georgia 2009

[192] Cancer Facts and Figures 2002 and 2003 www.cancer.org

[193] Campbell, TCC, *The China Study* pp51-65

[194] Karjalainen J, Martin JM, Knip M et al, "A bovine albumin peptide as a possible trigger of insulin-dependent Diabetes Mellitus," *NEJM*. 327 (1992):302-307

[195] Akerblom HK, Knip M. "Putative environmental factors and Type 1 diabetes." *Diabetes/Metabolism Revs* 14 (1998):31-67

[196] Naik RG and Palmer JP. "Preservation of beta-cell function in Type-1 Diabetes." *Diabetes Rev.* 7 (1999):154-182

[197] http://www.diabetes.org/diabetes-basics/diabetes-statistics/

[198] American Diabetes Association. "Type 2 diabetes in children and adolescents." *Diabetes Care* 23 (2000):381-389

[199] Data from the 2007 National Diabetes Fact Sheet (the most recent year for which data is available)

[200] Himsworth HP. "Diet and the incidence of diabetes mellitus." *Clin. Sci. 2* (1935):117-148

[201] Snowdon DA and Phillips RL. "Does a vegetarian diet reduce the occurrence of diabetes?" *Am. J. Publ. Health* 75 (1985):507-512

[202] Tsunehara CH, Leonetti, DL and Fujimoto WY. "Diet of second generation Japanese-American men with and without non-insulin dependent diabetes." *Am. J. Clin. Nutr.* 52 (1990):731-738

[203] Anderson JW. "Dietary fiber in nutrition management of diabetes." *In:* G. Vahouny, V and D Kritchevsky (eds), *Dietary Fiber: Basic and Clinical Aspects."* Pp.343-360. New York: Plenum Press,1986.

[204] Neal Barnard, M.D. et al, "A Low-Fat Vegan Diet Improves Glycemic Control and Cardiovascular Risk Factors in a Randomized Clinical Trial in Individuals With Type-2 Diabetes." *Diabetes Care* 29:1777-1783 1006 DOI: 10.2357/dc06-0606

[205] Neal Barnard, M.D. et al, "Changes in Nutrient Intake and Dietary Quality Among Participants With Type 2 Diabetes Following a Low-Fat Vegan Diet or a Conventional Diet for 22 Weeks." *J Am Dietetic Assoc.* October 2008 vol 108 #10;1636-1645

[206] Dahl-Jorgensen K, Joner G and Hanssen KF. "Relationship between cow's milk consumption and incidence of IDDM in childhood." *Diabetes Care* 14 (1991):1081-1083.

[207] Irizarry MC. Multiple Sclerosis. In: Cudkowicz ME, Irizarry MC, eds. *Neurologic Disorders in Women.* Boston, Ma: Butterworth–Heinemann; 1997:85

[208] Swank RL. "Effect of low saturated fat diet in early and late cases of multiple sclerosis." *Lancet* 336 (1990):37-39

[209] Swank RL. "Effect of low saturated fat diet in early and late cases of multiple sclerosis." *Lancet* 336 (1990):37-39

[210] Swank RL. "Treatment of multiple sclerosis with low fat diet." *A.M.A.Arch. Neurol. Psychiatry* 69 (1953):91-103

[211] Swank RL, and Bourdillon RB. "Multiple sclerosis: assessment of treatment with modified low fat diet." *J. Nerv. Ment. Dis.* 131 (1960):468-488

[212] Swank RL. "Multiple sclerosis: twenty years on low-fat diet." *Arch. Neurol.* 23 (1970):460-474

[213] Malosse D, Perron H, Sasco A, et al. "Correlation between milk and dairy product consumption and multiple sclerosis prevalence: a worldwide study." *Neuroepidemiology* 11 (1992):304-312

[214] Munari L, Lovati R, Boiko A. Therapy with glatiramer acetate for multiple sclerosis. Cochrane Database Syst Rev. 2004;(1):CD004678.

[215] Filippini G, Munari L, Incorvaia B, Ebers GC, Polman C, D'Amico R, Rice GP. Interferons in relapsing remitting multiple sclerosis: a systematic review. Lancet. 2003 Feb 15;361(9357):545-52.

[216] Clegg A, Bryant J. Immunomodulatory drugs for multiple sclerosis: a systematic review of clinical and cost effectiveness. Expert Opin Pharmacother. 2001 Apr;2(4):623-39.

[217] Guarner F, Malagelada JR. "Gut flora in health and disease." *Lancet.* 2003 Feb 8;361(9356):512-9.

[218] Peltonen R, Ling WH, Hanninen O, Eerola E. "An uncooked vegan diet shifts the profile of human fecal microflora: computerized analysis of direct stool sample gas-liquid chromatography profiles of bacterial cellular fatty acids." *Appl Environ Microbiol.* 1992 Nov;58(11):3660-6.

[219] Cashman KD, Shanahan F. "Is nutrition an aetiolgical factor in inflammatory bowel disease?" *Eur J. Gastroenterol. Hepatol* 15 no 6 June 2003:607-13

[220] Sakamoto N, et al, Epidemiology Group of the Research Committee on Inflammatory Bowel Disease in Japan "Dietary risk factors for inflammatory bowel disease: a multicenter case-control study in Japan." *Inflamm. Bowel Dis.* 11 no 2 February 2005:154-63

221 Magee E, "A nutritional component to inflammatory bowel disease: the contribution of meat to fecal sulfide excretion." *Nutrition* 15, no 3 March 1999:244-46

222 Truelove S. "Ulcerative colitis provoked by milk." *Br. Med. J.* 1961 1:154

223 Samuelsson SM. "Risk factors for extensive ulcerative colitis and ulcerative proctitis: a population based case-control study." *Gut* 32 no 12 December 1991:1526-30.

224 Wright R. "A controlled therapeutic trial of various diets in ulcerative colitis." *Br. Med J.* 1965 22:138-41

225 Jones VA, "Crohn's Disease: Maintenance of Remission by Diet." *Lancet* 2 no 8448 July 1985: 177-80

226 http://www.americanpregnancy.org/main/statistics.html

227 http://www.cdc.gov/ART/ART2005/index.htm

228 http://www.cdc.gov/ART/ART2005/index.htm

229 Chavarro, Jorge E et al, "Increasing adherence to a specific dietary pattern associated with a substantially reduced risk of infertility due to ovulation disorders," *Obstet Gynecol* 2007 110:1050-1058

230 Chavarro, et al, "Protein intake and ovulatory infertility," *Am J Obste Gynecol* 2008;198(2):210.el-7

231 Chavarro, Dr. Jorge, "A prospective study of dairy foods intake and anovulatory infertility," Feb 28 *Human Reproduction* doi:10.1093/humrep/demo19

232 "Asthma at a Glance," National Center for Environmental Health (NCEH), U.S. CDC, 1999

233 "Chronic Conditions: A Challenge for the 21st Century," National Academy on an Aging Society, 2000

234 "Morbidity and Mortality Report," NCHS, U.S. CDC, 2003

235 "The Costs of Asthma," Asthma and Allergy Foundation 1992 and 1998 2000 update

[236] "Morbidity and Mortality Weekly Report," Surveillance for Asthma, U.S. CDC, 2002

[237] Bealsey, R. "Worldwide variation in prevalence of symptoms of asthma, allergic rhinoconjunctivitis, and atopic eczema: ISAAC" *The Lancet*, Volume 351, Issue 9111, Pages 1225 - 1232, 25 April 1998 doi:10.1016/S0140-6736(97)07302-9

[238] Worldwide variation in prevalence of symptoms of asthma, allergic rhinoconjunctivitis, and atopic eczema: ISAAC Prof Richard Beasley, The International Study of Asthma and Allergies in Childhood (ISAAC) Steering Committee

[239] Sampson HA. "Update on Food allergy. Part 1: immunopathogenesis and clinical disorders." *J Allergy Clin Immunol.* 2004;113:805–819.

[240] Host A. "Frequency of cow's milk allergy in childhood." *Ann Allergy Asthma Immunol.* 2002;89(6 Suppl 1):33-7.

[241] Gunnbjörnsdóttir MI, Omenaas, E. et al. on behalf of the RHINE study group. "Obesity and nocturnal gastro-oesophageal reflux are related to onset of asthma and respiratory symptoms." *Eur Respir J* 2004; 24:116-121

[242] Barbas, AS, Downing TE et al. "Chronic aspiration shifts the immune response from Th1 to Th2 in a murine model of asthma." *Eur. J. Clin. Invest.* Volume 38 Issue 8, Pages 596 – 602 Published Online: 17 Jul 2008

[243] Salpeter, S, Buckley, N, et al. "Meta-Analysis: Effect of Long-Acting β-Agonists on Severe Asthma Exacerbations and Asthma-Related Deaths." *Ann Intern Med* June 20, 2006 144:904-912

[244] Lindahl O, Lindwall L, Spangberg A, Stenram A, Ockerman PA. "Vegan regimen with reduced medication in the treatment of bronchial asthma." *J Asthma* 1985;22:45-55.

[245] http://www.chiro.org/Wilk/

[246] Kemper et al, "Herbs and other dietary supplements: healthcare professional knowledge, attitude and practices," *Altern Ther Health Med* 2003;9:42-49

247 Cashman, et al, ""Massachusetts Registered Dietitians knowledge, attitude, personal use, and recommendations to clients about herbal supplements," *J Altern Complement Med* 203;9:735-746

248 Winslow, et al, "Physicians want education about complementary and alternative medicine to enhance communication with their patients," *Arch Intern Med* 2002;162:1176-1181

249 Stroupe KT, Morrison DA, Hlatky MA, et al. Investigators of Veterans Affairs Cooperative Studies Program #385 (AWESOME: Angina With Extremely Serious Operative Mortality Evaluation). Cost-effectiveness of coronary artery bypass grafts versus percutaneous coronary intervention for revascularization of high-risk patients. *Circulation.* 2006 Sep 19;114(12):1251-7.

250 American Diabetes Association "Economic Costs of Diabetes in the U.S. in 2007"

251 Munari, L, Lovati R, Boiko A "Therapt with glatiramer acetate for multiple sclerosis." Cochrane Database Syst Rev. 2004; (1):CD004678

252 Kobelt, G "Costs and Quality of Life in Multiple Sclerosis: A Cross Sectional Study in the USA."

253 Widley, et al, "Fat and sugar levels are high in snacks purchased from student stores in middle schools, *J Am Diet Assoc.* 2000; 100:319-322

254 Food Research and Action Center, "State of the States, 2005: A Profile of Food and Nutrition Programs across the Nation" (www.frac.org [March 22, 2005].

255 J. B. Schwimmer, T. M. Burwinkle, and J. W. Varni, "Health-Related Quality of Life of Severely Obese Children and Adolescents," *JAMA* 289, no. 14 (2003): 1813–19; A.

256 M. Tershakovec, S. C. Weller, and P. R. Gallagher, "Obesity, School Performance and Behaviour of Black, Urban Elementary School Children," *International Journal of Obesity & Related Metabolic Disorders* 18, no. 5 (1994): 323–27.

257 L. Parker, *The Relationship between Nutrition and Learning: A School Employee's Guide to Information and Action* (Washington: National Education Association, 1989)

258 Action for Healthy Kids, *The Learning Connection: The Value of Improving Nutrition and Physical Activity in Our Schools*, 2004 (www.ActionForHealthyKids.org [July 7, 2005]

259 308,124,465 population of U.S.
http://www.census.gov/main/www/popclock.html